Pain's
Healing
Secret

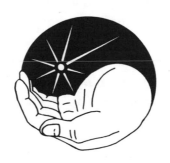

A Mystery Disease

Completely invisible
yet powerful, it holds
exhausted victims hostage
for months or years at a time.

It keeps them from what they love,
yet when they seek help,
willing to try anything to make it stop,
others believe they are not telling the truth.

Alone they believe they cannot change
the terrible thing happening
and when others cannot stop it
they feel helpless.

Rare in Eastern cultures,
yet common in the West,
it will not kill them,
but many die trying to break free.

Only recently have a majority of doctors recognized
— — — — — — — — — — — as a serious disease in the
United States.

Pain's Healing Secret

By Michael Turk

Illustrated by Alisse Suess

Edited with Brenda Hamilton

Acu Press

1551 Palm Avenue

Chico, California 95926

The excerpts from *The Man with the Miraculous
Hand*s by Joseph Kessel, translated by Helen
Weaver and Leo Raditsa, copyright 1961 by
Farrar, Straus and Cudhay, New York, were
originally published in France by Gillimard as
"Les Mains du Miracle" and are reprinted by
permission.

To my parents

Dad helped me know wonder

Mom taught me to sing and dance in my heart

Contents

List of Tables

Foreword

Mayama Morehart, M.D.

Finally a book on a safe and effective way to relieve pain! Nonprofessionals as well as physicians will find easy to understand, in-depth advice concerning the prevention of disease and the rapid healing of injuries.

In the Far East people have traditionally looked to nature for a cure. Michael Turk describes how natural healing methods have been used to promote longer healthier lives. His lucid descriptions empower the reader to use one's own energy to heal injuries and common diseases. Michael has studied ancient Chinese classics, and in the process has uncovered simple tools and forgotten principles of healing. Using this book, the reader can apply the ancient secrets of Oriental doctors right in their own home. Michael Turk explains how massage and acupressure can be used to stop pain and increase energy without the side effects of stimulants and drugs. The reader will learn how to feel energized, look younger and improve overall health.

Touch and massage strengthen the immune system and have been proven effective in the prevention of disease. Acupressure massage promotes the rapid healing of injuries and helps avoid complications. It can also reduce pain in chronically ill patients. On the other hand, the use of drugs may lead to further injuries by masking symptoms.

This book is a treasury of health secrets discovered in ancient medical classics. Michael has researched the hidden wisdom found in ancient Chinese acupoint names and medical terms. The reader is encouraged to explore these acupoints, releasing natural healing energy hidden below the skin. Included is advice about the best methods to restore the flow of energy. No other book explains so clearly and in such simple terms how to promote awareness of healing energy in the body. These health secrets have been proven practical through centuries of treating people with difficult problems. Michael shares these principles with those eager to help themselves and others.

Michael Turk has studied Asian medicine for more than thirty years and has taught classes for more than thirty-five years. He illustrates the text with inspiring stories drawn from his years of teaching and practicing *Shiatzu* massage. This book demystifies complex ancient terminology, which reveals long-held secrets of Oriental physicians.

Michael's painstaking research has produced a well-documented book, one that is appealing to a wide variety of readers. I highly recommend this book to those curious about energy healing. I especially recommend this book to those seeking health.

Preface

I had health problems all my life until I discovered Chinese medicine. In high school my favorite subjects were science and math. My first career was in electronics. I feel the benefits of disciplined scientific thinking have most directly benefitted my intellectual development. However, I nearly died three times, and though I had good doctors who saved my life, I was told my problems could not be corrected by medical science. My career path changed because these serious health crises left me weak and prone to illness. I had colds, flu and allergies nine months out of the year.

My wife Susan took up Japanese macrobiotic cooking and three months later I noticed, to my surprise, I had not been sick. After one particularly strenuous hike a year later, it dawned on me why kids like to run and play so hard! Asian medicine didn't make sense logically and was unproven scientifically, but it worked. The quality of my health and life improved dramatically. I studied macrobiotics to understand why. In my quest for understanding I discovered acupressure and was amazed at the way it excelled in relieving pain and increasing energy. I studied a type of acupressure massage called Shiatzu. After about ten years of teaching in the evening and helping friends, I decided to help fix people rather than electronic machines.

Gradually I began to see that science is one way of looking at and learning about the world, but traditional ways of knowing also had value. Jesus said, "You shall know them by their fruits" (Matthew 7:16). If you sample the fruits of traditional ways, you too can determine their true value.

I studied and applied traditional Chinese medicine until I discovered how to make the principles work. They worked

-16

for me, and I have been experiencing superior health ever since. I try here to clearly relate how to use these principles. If you don't try you'll never know.

February 14, 2001

Chico, California

Acknowledgments

The original idea for this book occurred in 1980 when Bill Mueller, who employed me as a *Shiatzu* massage instructor, asked me to put together some instructional material. My first editor, Nan VanGelder, changed my life forever when she showed me how beautiful it was to turn ideas into written words. With her help, a forty-page handbook titled *Shiatzu* was published in 1982.

Many students have helped me by taking great notes and giving me copies. The ones I can remember are Doug Bird, Mo Dewhurst, Valerie Swartz, Loren Lewison and Joane Rahiser.

Many friends have helped with the production of this book including Kris Kopping, Lani Lila, Lori Adams, Delina Fuchs, Jan Schmidl and Greg Catanese.

I first learned of *Shiatzu* in 1970, while studying with Michio Kushi, who educated and entertained me during his lectures. The inspired teaching of Shizuko Yamamoto, author of *Barefoot Shiatzu*, introduced me to *Shiatzu*. She could change pain into energy with a touch. In 1971 my next massage teacher, Bud Estes (longtime president of the American Judo and Jujitsu Foundation), taught me the strength in being gentle. It always amazed me to see this powerful martial artist gracefully move around on the floor combating his students' pain. He lived so compassionately that his spirit guides many of his students even now. I'm grateful for the help and friendship of Jacques de Langre author of *Do-in* who, in 1971 taught me Do-in Self Massage. In 1972 I took a class in traditional Oriental medicine from Naboru Muramoto, author of *Healing Ourselves*.

My heartfelt thanks to Arynne Simon, who taught me to express myself assertively.

I wish to thank Joey Lazaro, director of the California Acupuncture College, who put up with me as a student and teacher.

My humble thanks to Henry Chueng, an herbalist who took me under his wing and taught me about Chinese herbs and encouraged me to write this book.

Finally, editing with Brenda has been a labor of laughter.

Introduction

    People are often surprised when I show them how easy it is to relieve pain. The purpose of *Pain's Healing Secret* is to enable you to relieve pain by stimulating a healing response that feels like energy and speeds the healing of disease and injuries. My goal in writing this book is to empower people who are suffering from pain to heal the cause of their suffering and to teach others to help those who are suffering from pain. Acupressure cannot always cure disease, but it can relieve pain, reduce the need for pain pills, increase energy and improve resistance to disease.

    What is pain? Is pain an emotion like fear, anger and love? Is pain a sensation like hot, cold and sharp? Is pain located in the body or centered in the mind? Is pain punishment for past mistakes? (Pain is used to train and is often used to torture.) Is pain an experience or a memory? Is pain a symptom of disease? Is pain a warning or does it have no meaning? One answer to the question, "What is pain?" is hidden in an ancient Asian medical book and inspired the development of acupuncture and acupressure.

    What is a secret? A secret is knowing something that others do not know. Secret knowledge is kept a mystery by some people to wield power over others. Today many ancient secrets and mysteries are coming to light, yet pain is still a mystery. The solution to a mystery is a secret. Acupuncture has been scientifically demonstrated to relieve pain. What is the secret to the success of acupuncture in relieving pain? Many secrets will be revealed about pain, disease and traditional Chinese medicine in this book.

    What you think about pain can hurt you.

This book exposes modern myths about pain and reveals methods of relieving pain that have proven effective for hundreds of years. Actually this knowledge has been in writing for over two millennia. One of the strange truths about pain is: the more pain pills are used, the less effective they become. Consequently, when the dose is increased, or stronger and more expensive drugs are used, there is a greater risk of side effects, including more pain. This effect is called rebound pain. Ultimately, masking pain makes it worse. A Chinese proverb warns, "Before you shoot a dog learn its owner's name." If you need to take pain pills you should ask your doctor's advice about using acupressure to cut down on unnecessary drugs.

The world-renowned hand surgeon, leprosy expert and pain researcher, Dr. Paul Brand, has written a sensitive book about his experiences with those suffering from pain. He clearly explains how "numbing out" with drugs can injure tissue and create the need for more drugs. In *Pain: The Gift Nobody Wants*, he wrote, "Frantic attempts to silence pain signals may actually have a paradoxical effect" (pages 185–190).

Mass media has a knack for characterizing the interests of a generation. The hip generation got high only to discover they crashed and burned. They learned drugs used to stimulate energy resulted in depletion of energy. Others learned pain pills used to "numb out" led to pain, which required more pain pills.

Today, Generation Xers pursue energy, while the Baby Boomer generation seeks pain relief. The ongoing cultural exchange between Asia and America has much to offer both generations. Since World War II Asian martial arts have become popular as exercise because the arts emphasize awareness of personal energy. Recently, the effectiveness of Asian healing arts to relieve pain has become recognized by the National Institute of Health and the American Medical Association. Asian healing also uses energy. A common name for this type of healing is energetic medicine. These methods can be a part of anyone's basic health care at home.

For those who seek energy and want pain relief, two principles of energetic medicine apply. Food and herbs provide energy, while acupoint therapies direct energy. There are only two mistakes people make about energy. The first is failing to learn to control it while they are young, and the second is failing to learn to generate it when they are older. People are looking for complicated answers; they find it hard to believe a simple answer can be powerful. Most pain can be relieved by simple methods that move energy.

Some people intuitively know how to use energy for healing. Energetic medicine also can be learned. It is taught to students who spend years in acupuncture school. This book deals with a complicated and technical subject, but the simple truth found in the ancient medical classics is easy to understand and use. Pain and energy are related. Pain is injured energy. Pain goes when energy flows.

This book is organized as follows:

The Experience of Pain chapter discusses pain and how it affects people's lives. Various ideas about pain are considered, including a curious ancient Chinese idea that pain is injured energy. The Chinese word *Qi* (here translated as energy) is used in everyday spoken Chinese in ways that may surprise non-Chinese speaking people.

All you need to know to relieve most pain and increase energy is explained in **The Experience of Qi Energy** chapter. It describes how people experience *Qi* energy and teaches how this power can be used to heal pain. These methods can be used today to relieve many types of pain and speed the healing of injuries. The exercises are given to help you experience the *Qi* energy that relieves pain.

The chapter on **Ancient Asia** traces the ideas of Asian healing in Chinese medical writing back to the dawn of Chinese civilization. This chapter attempts to separate myth from history. You will meet fascinating folks who made history, conceived the ideas and wrote the books revered by many modern Chinese and practitioners of traditional Chinese medicine.

The **Traditional Chinese Medicine** chapter takes a deeper look at the idea of *Qi* energy in Chinese medical writing, following how it spread to other Asian countries. Other curious theories about health, symptoms and disease are mentioned as well as other methods of healing. The yinyang theory and its application to health and disease is introduced.

The **Change Pain into Energy** section introduces terms and concepts specific to the Oriental ideas about the origin, progression and transformation of pain in the body. A method of evaluating pain and the energy response is presented. The yinyang theory is used to evaluate the depth, color (appearance) and quality of pain using easily observed signs and commonly experienced symptoms.

The *Shiatzu* **Movements** section illustrates four easy-to-learn massage methods that produce benefits far greater than the effort to perform them. A section on acupoint basics briefly defines acupoint and *meridian* terminology used in this book.

The **Four Acupoints for a Healthy Self** chapter provides detailed information to easily locate four of the most frequently used acupoints. These are the most powerful acupoints that change pain into energy. Knowledge of these points can be applied daily to warn of health problems and to release energy for pain relief, healing and stress reduction. For the last two millennia, sage healers have praised these points.

The **Eight More to Heal Thyself** chapter describes additional acupoints that relieve pain and symptoms of common ailments. These acupoints are easy to find on yourself and provide additional benefits to the immune system and the brain.

The **Sixteen Acupoints for a Partner to Press** chapter details more very powerful acupoints you may press by yourself to relieve pain and provide additional health benefits, but they are located in out-of-the-way places. This means it's easier if you have a study buddy to press your buttons.

The ***Shiatzu* Session** chapter gives suggestions about how to perform the art of *Shiatzu* massage. It includes how to prepare for a session, precautions to observe and a *Shiatzu* routine, listing the points and locations in logical order.

The **Acupressure Therapy** chapter lists common health problems and the points most likely to bring relief.

The **Fuxi's Biography by Confucius** (appendix) found in the *I Ching* is the most extensive information surviving from the ancient past.

The **Yellow Sovereign on the Cause of Pain** (appendix) is the first twenty percent of chapter five of *The Yellow Sovereign's Classic of Internal Medicine (Huangdi Neijing, Suwen* 黃 帝 內 經 素 問) titled "Grand Theory on the Reciprocal Nature of Yinyang" *(Yinyang Yingxiang Dalun* 陰 陽 應 像 大 論). Included is the theory on the cause of pain.

The **Inductive and Deductive Logic** (appendix) is an essay on logic for those who would like to understand more about the difference between relational thinking and rational thinking.

The **Glossary of Terms** (in English and in *Pinyin)* lists terms introduced in the text, including pronunciation and definitions.

Recommended Reading and **Recommended Schools** are for those who would like to know more about this ancient art.

The **Bibliography** has some of the author's favorite books that inspired or provided information for this book.

The **Afterword** is just that.

The **Index** includes people, places and things mentioned in the text.

Notice

This book is written with both the professional and the beginner in mind. If you are new to energy work, first read it quickly, then read it again slowly for understanding. It's okay not to understand everything the first time through.

Warning—Disclaimer

Do not use drugs while operating your energy equipment. This book introduces the reader to an Asian theory of biological energy as understood by modern practitioners of acupuncture, acupressure massage and traditional Chinese medicine. Studies have shown that both legal and illegal psychoactive drugs inhibit nerve responses required for these methods to work. If your nerves have been damaged or suppressed or you need drugs to control pain, seek the advice of your doctor.

If you are currently on prescribed medication, it is recommended you consult your physician before making any changes. It is always a good idea to inform your doctor when using alternative medicine. He/she may help you be certain that you not only feel well but that your prognosis has improved. It's best not only to feel good but also to be able to do more with less effort. Ask your doctor's help in cutting down on unnecessary medications. A professional acupressure therapist or an acupuncturist may be able to provide therapy for damaged nerves.

This book is sold with the understanding that by publishing this book the author is not engaged in rendering medical or other professional services. If you need medical or other expert assistance, the services of a licensed acupuncturist, chiropractor or medical professional should be sought. This book is about maintaining and regaining health so disease will disappear.

Use the best of East and West. "It takes more than one pillar to hold up a temple," advises an ancient Chinese saying, and "A smart doctor does not treat himself." Using acupressure, acupuncture, chiropractic in conjunction with standard medical procedures can benefit most health problems.

It is not the purpose of this book to cover all the information otherwise available, but to complement, amplify and supplement other texts. You are urged to read all available material, learn as much as possible about your energy system and tailor the information to your individual needs. For more information, see the additional reading section and the bibliography.

Acupressure is not a cure-all. Some health problems are relieved entirely while others can't be helped at all. Plan on taking time to learn all you can about your health problems, including modern medical understanding of the human body and standard Red Cross first aid.

Every effort has been made to make this book as complete and accurate as possible. However, there may be mistakes both typographical and in content. Therefore, this text should be used only as a general guide and not as the ultimate source of information on pain and health. Furthermore, this book contains information on the acupuncture energy system as understood by the author. As new information becomes available, the ideas and facts expressed in this book may change.

The purpose of this book is to educate and entertain. The publisher, Acu Press and the author shall have neither liability nor responsibility to any person or entity with respect to any loss or damage caused or alleged to be caused, directly or indirectly by the information contained in this book. If you find errors or omissions in this book you are urged to write the author so future editions may be accurate. Write to Acu Press, P. O. Box 7527, Chico, California 95927 or e-mail to acupress@learnacupressure.com.

How to Use This Book

For those in pain who want quick relief read **The Experience of *Qi* Energy** chapter, which provides the basic information on eliminating unwanted pain. This may be all the information you need; however, additional points are listed in the **Acupressure Therapy** chapter. If additional location information is needed, read about the acupoint in the body of the text. Use the index or table of contents to find the acupoint. For those interested in a whole-body *Shiatzu* massage see the chapter **A *Shiatzu* Session**.

This book can be read in any order. Feel free to jump around and use the glossary and index to acquaint yourself with unfamiliar terms.

Chinese Language Conventions in this Book

The Chinese language is very different from English in many ways. This book explores some of those differences to help in the understanding of the Chinese way of thinking, which developed a different approach to health care and has proven to be very successful in relieving pain.

Most languages consist of a spoken and a written aspect. The Chinese language is unique in both aspects. The written language contains images combined to express ideas referred to as ideographic. The People's Republic of China has simplified the complex images in the written language to make it easier to learn and write, but the traditional written characters are more expressive and are used exclusively in this book.

The Chinese spoken language contains words that sound similar except for the tone which can rise, fall, dip or remain level as a particular word is spoken. We use tone to change the meaning of a word in subtle ways. Consider the word "no," for example, in a conversation as a photographer prepares to take a traveler's passport photo. The photographer asks, "Are you ready?" The traveler simply says, "No (monotone)." As she prepares for the photo, she smiles. The photographer says, "Don't smile." The traveler questions "No (rising tone)?" The photographer says emphatically, "No (falling tone)!" The traveler queries, "No (tone drops then rises), why not?" The photographer replies, "You can't smile on passport photos."

The Chinese spoken language uses tone to indicate entirely different words. Many different written characters use the sound huang: 'agitated (慌)' uses huang1 (level tone), 'yellow (黄)' uses huang2 (rising tone), 'lie (謊)' uses huang3 (tone drops then rises), 'shake, sway (晃)' uses huang4 (falling tone). Furthermore, very different written characters can use the same sound and tone. Huang (rising tone) means 'yellow (黄)' or 'sage-king (皇)' depending on the sound that accompanies it. Thus, Huanghe (黄河) means the 'Yellow River' and huangdi (皇帝) means 'emperor.' On rare occasions, two polysyllable words will have the same sound and tone pattern, in which case the context indicates the meaning when spoken. It is, however, usually not an accident that the words are identical.

Pinyin was developed by the People's Republic of China to aid non-Chinese in pronunciation. *Pinyin* is very helpful when learning Chinese terminology, but many people new to the convention find it confusing. This book has pronunciation 'helps' (sounds like "hell+pss") to approximate the way Chinese is spoken by English speakers who usually do not learn the tones. The 'helps' are similar to children's word games wherein pictures and letters are used to make phrases. When there is a (+), run the sounds together; when there is a space, the sounds are each distinctive (sounds like "dis tink tiv"). When the word is capitalized, pronounce the word as a personal name. Lower case words are as they sound in American (sounds like "ah Mary kin") English. Capitalized single letters are pronounced as letters of the alphabet in American English (sounds like "E+ng glish").

Chinese personal names are written in the classical Chinese way with sir names first and given names last. This is the opposite way personal names are written in the West, except on forms that instruct: last name first (one of the many differences between the East and the West pointed out in this book).

Conventions Specific to this Book

Chinese words and terms in this book are accompanied by traditional Chinese characters, Chinese *Pinyin*, a literal translation, easy to understand English and/or pronunciation 'helps.' This book contains many specific ideas and terms that may be new to some readers. In order to aid in understanding, the following conventions have been established:

technical terms (italics) for traditional Chinese medical terms

PINYIN (all caps) for the transliteration of Chinese words

TECHNICAL TERMS in PINYIN (italics, all caps) for traditional Chinese medical terms

Acupoint Nicknames (small caps) some old, some new, some coined by the author to identify acupoints

"Article Titles" (double quotes) for modern publications

Book and *Movie Title*s (italics) for ancient and modern texts

BOOK TITLES in *PINYIN* (italics capitalized) for ancient Chinese texts

Names in Pinyin (capitalized) for Chinese names

"Quotations" (double quotes) for direct quotes

'concepts' (single quotes) for conceptual designations

emphasis (bold)

(clarifying comments) (parentheses)

-date means before the common era in preference to B.C.

+date means common era in preference to A.D.

b. = birth, d. = death

Chinese characters used are ancient (called traditional) rather than modern (called simplified)

The body inch (寸 CUN) is a unit of measurement unique to each body

Meridians are named after internal organs and energy systems. Acupoints are named after *meridians* and given a serial number. An abbreviated acupoint identifier is used in this text. It is composed of a two-letter abbreviation of the *meridian* followed by a number (i.e., Gv.20).

A note on the spelling of *Shiatzu:* Japanese acupressure massage has been spelled both *Shiatsu* and *Shiatzu* since I began teaching. I obviously prefer the letter 'z,' the most neglected letter in the alphabet. As far as I can tell, the Japanese don't care either way. They don't use the Roman alphabet except on tee shirts because they think the Roman alphabet is exotic and looks cool.

Two thousand years ago the Japanese first adopted some ideographic Chinese characters to represent similar spoken words. Seven hundred years later they developed a unique phonographic writing system that could represent the rest of their spoken language. In Japan, *Shiatzu* can be written with the uniquely Japanese written glyphs or the Chinese characters (指壓).

The Experience of Pain

Chronic pain is only an abstract idea unless you have had persistent pain severe enough that you would try anything to make it stop. Unless you have endured pain agonizing enough that you had to keep moving by pacing or other avoidance behaviors to distract yourself, then horrible pain cannot be understood—even reason cannot bring understanding. Unless you have experienced pain intensely enough that your mind cannot focus, your brain stops working and you feel paralyzed, excruciating pain is beyond imagination. When someone tells you they have terrible pain, do you think they are exaggerating, trying to get sympathy, attention, or perhaps faking to get out of work? Do you suspect they have some other motive?

You were taught that pain is a sensation that protects you from injury, but when pain will not stop, then that warning system seems to be without meaning. You have heard and may accept "no pain, no gain," but this kind of pain has no gain, no reason. You are doing all you can do; the injury is healed. You desperately ask, "Why does it continue to hurt?" Painkilling drugs often lose their power to stop or reduce pain. Surgery cannot be performed when there is no problem. Can you imagine being told there is no reason for your pain?

You may have always recovered quickly with very little pain in order to resume your active life, but this pain will not stop; your life is on hold. Acute pain warns of an injury, it makes us slow down or stop to prevent further injury, but chronic pain seems to give a meaningless message. Strange how some diseases are accompanied by terrible pain, and other more serious diseases produce little or no pain. You know the reason for your pain, therefore, why does this pain go on without a purpose?

Perhaps you do not express your emotions well and were told the pain comes from bottling up your feelings. However, an emotional friend was told pain comes from emotions. If the pain is in your head, why do you feel it in your body?

You have just entered the mysterious world of pain. Western philosophers, poets, doctors and scientists are as baffled about pain as you may be.

Paul Brand, an eminent authority on pain, studied Western medicine in England, practiced medicine in India and directed research in the United States. He is a world-renowned hand surgeon and an expert on leprosy. His book, *Pain: The Gift Nobody Wants*, published in 1993, clearly states on page 187:

> My esteem for pain runs so counter to the common attitude that I sometimes feel like a subversive, especially in modern Western countries. On my travels I have observed an ironic law of reversal at work: as a society gains the ability to limit suffering, it loses the ability to cope with what suffering remains. (It is the philosophers, theologians, and writers of the affluent West, not the Third World, who worry obsessively about 'the problem of pain,' and point an accusing finger at God.)

One Third World culture that has maintained the ability to handle pain is the Chinese. Since ancient times, Chinese medicine has used acupressure massage to relieve pain.

Friend or Foe?

There emerged from the horrors of World War II an unlikely hero who has been all but forgotten. Felix Kersten, a socially admired doctor of massage, had a successful practice in several European capitals. He looked like a solid

Flemish burgermeister with his domed head, broad brow, kind blue eyes and sensual mouth. This easygoing, stout man loved the good things of life: art, food and beautiful women.

In 1921 Kersten received a degree in scientific massage in Finland where massage is a most respected art and science. He also studied in Berlin where he met Dr. Ko, a little old Chinese gentleman trained as a doctor by Tibetan monks who in turn taught him acupressure. This old method, new to Kersten, surprised him with its precision and wisdom. Dr. Ko taught him how to use his intuition to go to the cause of the problem. After three years of intensive study, Kersten inherited Dr. Ko's large practice. By 1928 Kersten was an established success, booked up for three months in advance. His reputation spread throughout the continent where he treated the elite of European society with acupressure.

In 1939 Dr. Kersten was presented with a dilemma. Being of a temperate and peaceful disposition, he had avoided politics until a respected friend asked him to examine Reichsführer Heinrich Himmler. It was no secret Himmler had health problems. He had suffered from crippling stomach pains for years without relief. When the best medical treatment available failed, his doctor recommended Kersten.

Kersten was repulsed by the idea, but this friend appealed to his good nature. He indicated it would be a great service to his friends who were in fear of Himmler's dreadful power, that it was his professional duty and pressed his point by asking that he do this as a personal favor.

Himmler had commanded the SS with its elite death squad, the Gestapo, since 1929. In 1934, one year after Hitler came to power, the former school master became Hitler's hangman when his hand-picked SS men cunningly trapped and assassinated Ernst Röehm, who commanded the storm troopers (called the SA or brown shirts) and twelve of his fellow officers, who threatened to overthrow Hitler.

By 1939, when Kersten met Himmler, he was the second most powerful man in the Third Reich. He directed all secret police, who spawned a climate of mistrust and treachery through surveillance, censored mail and interrogation. Later that year Hitler declared war, invaded Poland and launched the occupation of France, Belgium, Holland, Norway, Denmark, Yugoslavia and half of Eastern Europe. Himmler's name was connected with cruelty—with vileness. People were filled with loathing, terror and fear of Himmler and the secret police.

How interesting that chronic severe abdominal pain caused a man as powerful as Himmler to seek alternative medicine from a famous doctor of massage. Eventually, Himmler depended exclusively on Kersten to relieve his pain. Kersten used his pain relieving power to save the lives of countless numbers of people and changed the outcome of World War II.

Himmler was reported to have said to his subordinate, Walter Schellenberg, "With every one of his massages, Dr. Kersten deprives me of a life." This startling statement came out at the time of the Nürnberg trials. Schellenberg, the head of the Third Reich's Intelligence Agency, on trial for war crimes and trying to gain leniency, claimed he had influenced Himmler to spare the lives of seven Swedish businessmen. However, separate investigations revealed that Dr. Felix Kersten, Himmler's private doctor, had saved the lives of these businessmen in addition to thousands of other prisoners marked for execution, while he himself was virtually a captive.

At first, Dr. Kersten secretly received and sent messages to Dutch friends and used his influence to save their lives. Later, he boldly influenced Himmler to stop the deportation of millions of Dutch from Holland to Poland.

4

"... bending over Himmler in the attitude of a baker kneading dough, Kersten said with great force and gravity, 'This deportation is the greatest mistake of your career'" *(Man with the Miraculous Hands,* page 102). Kersten even persuaded Himmler to stop the diabolical policy of starving the occupied countries of France, Belgium, Finland and Holland, a policy used to punish the resistance, all the while asking Himmler, as personal favors, to stop many executions and release prisoners. At great risk, Dr. Kersten personally arranged for Himmler to meet with a representative of the World Jewish Organization to arrange for the release of five thousand Jews into the hands of the Swiss Red Cross.

Finally, near the end of the war, Hitler, now a madman and head of a dying regime, vowed to drag down millions of innocent people with him. Dr. Kersten appealed to Himmler's vanity and gratitude toward him to stop the madness. Hitler had ordered Himmler to dynamite the concentration camps and to bomb without warning the occupied Dutch capitol of The Hague. Hitler ordered, "This city of Germanic traitors must die before us, and to the last man." Dr. Kersten persuaded Himmler to disobey his idol, Adolf Hitler. On March 12, 1945, in the presence of Dr. Felix Kersten and his private secretary, the reichsführer signed what he himself called *A Contract in the Name of Humanity* which stopped the concentration camps from being dynamited, allowed packages to be sent to individual Jewish prisoners and stopped, without exception, the execution of all Jews. Two days later, after much pleading, he disobeyed the Fuhrer's orders to use V2 rockets to bomb The Hague. He caved in to Dr. Kersten saying, "You are right about The Hague. It is, after all, a Germanic city. I'll spare it. The city will raise the white flag and will be surrendered to the Allies."

How did this good doctor of massage, utterly opposed to Nazism and all it stood for, gain influence over the second most powerful leader of the Nazi party? What power allowed him to gradually control Hitler's hangman? Dr. Felix Kersten knew a secret: how to relieve pain.

The authorized biography entitled, *The Man with the Miraculous Hands*, written by Joseph Kessel, describes his first treatment with Himmler. Kersten began without asking a single question.

The fingers glided over the smooth skin. Their tips skimmed in turn over Himmler's throat, chest, heart, and stomach. At first their touch was light, barely perceptible. Then the antennae began to stop at certain spots, to press down, to seek, to listen. ...

(later in the treatment)

Suddenly, Himmler gave a cry. The fingers, up to now so light and velvety as they glided over the surface of his body, had just pressed brutally on a spot in the stomach from which the pain burst forth like a wave of fire.

"Very good ... hold still," said Kersten softly.

Under the pressure of his hand, another tongue of pain burned and ravaged Himmler's intestines. Then another, and still another. The reichsfuhrer groaned and chewed his lips. His brow was wet with perspiration.

"That is very painful, isn't it?" asked Kersten each time.

"Terribly," answered Himmler between clenched teeth.

(after the treatment)

Himmler raised his body slowly, carefully, as if it contained a priceless treasure. ... But his physical relief, the incomparable peace which follows the disappearance of unbearable pain, still remained.

Himmler fixed Kersten with a look which, behind the glass of the spectacles, revealed a kind of bewilderment.

"Am I dreaming? Is it possible? The pain is gone ... completely gone."

He caught his breath and went on, more to himself than to Kersten, "No medicine works. ... Even morphine has lost its effect ... and now, in a few minutes—No, I would never have believed it."

(The book continues.)

"Doctor," he said, "I want to keep you near me" (pages 53–57).

Hugh R. Trevor-Roper, a respected Oxford professor of history and a noted authority on German affairs during World War II, wrote in the preface of *Kersten's Memoirs* "... there is no man whose story has been subjected to such minute investigation. It has been weighed by scholars, jurists, and even by political opponents, and has triumphed over all these tests."

These excerpts from Dr. Kersten's biography reveal some little-known facts about the secrets of his success. Even when morphine fails to relieve pain, acupressure can. Pain has many secrets. Experienced acupressure therapists first examine the body for sensitive areas using light pressure. Next, using more pressure, they test tender spots to evaluate which are the most sensitive. There is "good" pain and "bad" pain, and a small amount of pain can relieve a greater pain. After intense pain is relieved, a pleasurable feeling remains. Scientists now know this peaceful feeling comes from our body's own mood-elevating pain relievers called endorphins.

The book *The Man with the Miraculous Hands* changed my life. After reading it I decided to learn massage and exchange massages with friends and an occasional professional. I wanted to do something more humanitarian than engineering, so I became a massage therapist.

Is pain a friend or a foe? There is a secret to keeping pain a friend rather than a foe: sometimes people start out as friends and become enemies later. Pain usually begins as a friend protecting you from serious injury or warning of excesses that can hurt you. Pain comes around like a co-dependent friend who helps when needed, but can become clingy if not given a firm hand. An ancient Chinese saying advises, "It is better for friends to visit than to move in and stay."

To summarize, pain can be used to locate, evaluate and relieve pain, which, once relieved, leaves a feeling of peaceful well-being. This may seem strange to some people, but not to those who have received therapeutic massage from an experienced practitioner. Pain can be an unwanted guest or a friend with truthful bitter words. You can accept bitter words from a friend. Other Chinese sayings suggest, "Bitter words are good medicine—sweet words carry infection," and, "Both jade and character are shaped with bitter tools."

What Is Pain?

Many books have been written over the millennia that address the question: what is pain? Below are a few references. The first definition of pain is taken from the acknowledged standard for the English language, *The Oxford English Dictionary (OED)*, followed by a chronological selection from different encyclopedias. Finally, we will reverse the order of references from the present back to ancient times seeking the opinions of various authorities.

The *Oxford English Dictionary* defines pain: "1: Suffering or loss inflicted for a crime or offense; punishment; penalty; a fine. 2: A primary condition of sensation or consciousness, the opposite of *pleasure*; the sensation which one feels when hurt (in body or mind); suffering, distress" *(OED.* 2nd edition on CD-ROM. +1992).

The complete entry on pain from the *Encyclopedia Britannica* +1771 first edition in three volumes reads, "PAIN, is defined to be an uneasy sensation arising from a sudden and violent solution of the continuity, or some other accident in the nerves, membranes, vessels, muscles, &c. of the body; or, according to some, it consists in a motion of the organs of sense; and, according to others, it is an emotion of the soul occasioned by these organs."

A four-paragraph entry on pain from the *Chambers's Encyclopedia* +1884 edition in six volumes includes, "... Pain differs not only in its character, which may be dull, sharp, aching, tearing, gnawing, stabbing, &c., but in its mode of occurrence; for example, it may be flying or persistent, intermittent, remittent, or continued. It is not always that the pain is felt in the spot where the cause of it exists."

A more recent entry from a twenty-three paragraph article on pain from the *Encyclopedia Britannica* +1999 edition in thirty-two volumes on CD-ROM states, "... Acute pain is generally the easiest to control, medication and rest being effective treatments. Some pain, however, may defy treatment and persist for years. This chronic pain can be compounded by the psychological effects of hopelessness and anxiety."

"Chronic pain, mysterious, dull, and nonfatal, might be called the defining illness of our low profile, private, safe-sexed, self-absorbed era," wrote David B. Morris in *The Culture of Pain* published +1991.

"We treat pain as a diagnosis, not a symptom," said Michael Kilbride, the founder of the new Pain Management Center at the Muskegon, Michigan, General Hospital, as quoted in the book *The Culture of Pain* published +1991.

"Evil being the root of mystery, pain is the root of knowledge," said Simone Weil (b. +1909, d. +1943), French philosopher and mystic, in *New York Notebook* written in +1942 and published in +1950.

"Much of your pain is self-chosen. It is the bitter potion by which the physician within you heals your sick self," prescribed Kahlil Gibran in *The Prophet* published +1923.

Pain is "the simple reaction, which physically is expressed as the Law of Self-conservation, psychically as the Principle of following Pleasure and avoiding Pain," wrote A. Barratt, a metaphysician, in *Physical Metempiric* published +1883.

"Nature has placed mankind under the governance of two masters, pain and pleasure," wrote Jerry Bentham (b. +1748, d. +1832), an English philosopher, economist and theoretical jurist. "Pleasure ... the only good. Pain ... the only evil."

"The honest man takes pains, and then enjoys pleasures; the knave takes pleasure, and then suffers pains," wrote the American rebel and inventor Benjamin Franklin (b. +1706, d. +1790) in his popular *Poor Richard's Almanack,* a calendar of astronomical information for farmers to guide in planting and harvesting that included advice on health, travel, success and humor.

"What is pain? Tis a sensation produced on the tension of a nerve. ... But unto the man that is chastened with pain. ... Think; alas, what have my sins procured!" decreed Cotton Mather, (b. +1663, d. +1728), in his book on medicine *The Angel of Bethesda* which mixed religion with medicine and represented Europe's advanced science of the day.

"One word frees us of all the weight and pain of life. That word is love," wrote Sophocles in *Oedipus at Colonus,* -406.

"Pain is injured *Qi,*" stated the Yellow Sovereign, an ancient Chinese sage, in chapter 5, "The Grand Theory of the Reciprocal Nature of Yinyang" *(Yinyang Yingxiang Dalun* 陰陽應像大論 circa -4th century Chinese medical classic titled, *Huangdi Neijing, Suwen* 黃帝内經素問).

What Is *Qi*?

The Yellow Sovereign said pain is injured *Qi* (氣 sounds like "chee"), but what is *Qi*? *Qi* has the everyday meaning of weather, air, breath, vapor or vitality. In Chinese philosophy and medicine it represents the energy of nature or the life force. China's ancient sages conceived of an invisible energy that animates all forms of matter causing movement or

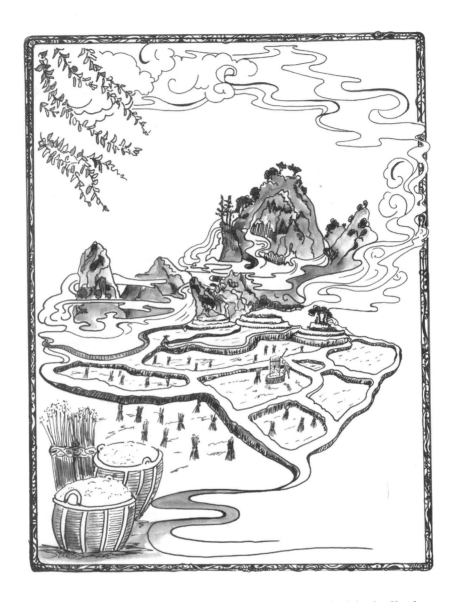

change. It is the principle of development behind all phenomena.

The written word *Qi* originated as an ideograph. The ancient Chinese character for *Qi* is the image of vapor 气 above rice 米. Scenes of vapor hanging in the air over rice paddies must have been a common sight for those ancient scribes who lived in the Yellow River flood basin. Viewing the early morning or evening haze that forms in layers over the surface of lakes and paddies suggests the idea of air and weather. Yearly floods made the soil rich which was ideal for farming. The Chinese sculpted the land into irrigated rice paddies. Early human beings cultivated the earth and from necessity, they reordered their lives creating fertile ground for cultivating ideas.

Agriculture created the need for record keeping and calendars, thus making it possible to know when to plant, when to harvest and when to prepare for the yearly flood. A record of the amount of grain harvested and used by the community made it possible to plan next year's harvest, market the surplus and impose taxes. In the beginning, written symbols helped folks remember images and record ideas. Later written records improved communication over great distances and endowed the gift of knowledge with a long life.

A Chinese written character is composed of one or more images, which represent an object or an abstract idea. Objects are usually represented by a graphic image sketched with brush strokes. Abstract ideas are usually represented by an arrangement of images within the character, suggesting an abstract concept or that which cannot be seen. Air, weather, breath and the life force are invisible or abstract ideas embraced by the word *Qi*. The image of vapor above rice can be said to represent the air above a rice paddy made visible because of the humidity. Other explanations for this character have been suggested over the centuries. Later, another possible explanation will be examined. The image of vapor above a rice paddy can be extended to include the weather particularly important to farming. The image of vapor also suggests smoky breath on a frosty day. Stretching the image further, the breath of life represents the life force.

The character *Qi* has a wide range of meanings. It is usually used with other characters to distinguish in which sense it is meant. Over the millennia philosophers and scientists in China have used this character to form terms, which rep-

12

resent specific complex ideas associated with what we today refer to as the life force.

Qi Used in Modern Chinese

Word	*Image*	*Spoken*	*Character*
air	space *Qi*	KONGQI	空氣
anger	produce *Qi*	SHENGQI	生氣
asthma	*Qi* wheeze	QICHUAN	氣喘
breath	*Qi* interest	QIXI	氣息
Chinese yoga	*Qi* effect(iveness)	QIGONG	氣功
complexion	*Qi* color	QISE	氣色
exhale	exit *Qi*	CHUQI	出氣
inhale	inspire *Qi*	XIQI	吸氣
strength	*Qi* power	QILI	氣力
temperament	spleen *Qi*	PIQI	脾氣
vigor	original *Qi*	YUANQI	元氣
weather	heaven *Qi*	TIANQI	天氣

The ancient Chinese identified many types of *Qi*. For example, during intercourse, the conception of a living being results when the father's *Essential Qi* (*JINGQI* 精氣 sounds like "jeeng chee") combines with the mother's *Essential Qi* (*JINGQI*). At this time the new being receives a lifetime of *Essential Qi*. Finally, when this *Essential Qi* is depleted, natural death occurs. Quality *Essential Qi* endows a person with strength, skill and dexterity to perform great feats effortlessly. When teaching the arts of China, especially the martial arts, training to develop *JINGQI* was included in the disciplines. This same *Essential Qi* starts the *Original Qi* (vigor *YUANQI* 元氣 sounds like you+ahn chee) flowing, which flows around the body for the life of the individual. *Qi* can be replenished with proper diet and *Qi* exercises. *Food Qi* (*GUQI* 穀氣 sounds like "goo chee") acquired from eating and *Air Qi* (*KONGQI* 空氣 sounds like "kong chee") acquired from breathing combine with *Essential Qi* to produce

Healthy Qi (upright ZHENGQI 正氣 sounds like "jeng chee"), the energy for healing and the ability to prevent disease.

However, an excess of normally beneficial *Qi* or an excess of harmful *Qi* will unbalance the *Healthy Qi* which results in disease. For example, extremes of weather *(Heaven Qi)* can cause diseases like the common cold or other upper respiratory infections. Additionally, overexposure to the elements can cause a heat stroke or frostbite. Also, excesses or deficiencies in diet disturb the balance of *Qi* stored in the organs. The theories of traditional Chinese medicine propose more than thirty different types of *Qi* to explain how the muscles, *blood*, immune system, *internal* organs, mind and emotions can acquire, store or use *Qi* energy.

To summarize the theory of *Qi*, disease results from an excess or deficiency of internal *Qi* and/or a disruption of circulating external *Qi*. If you have good inner *Qi*, you will have health and vitality.

"Anxiety retards the movement of *Qi*" (teachings from *Root Spirit*, chapter 8 *Ben Shen* 本神 of the *Huangdi Neijing, Lingshu* 黄帝内經靈樞).

"Anger raises *Qi*, ... pleasure relaxes *Qi*, ... grief dissolves *Qi*, ... fear drops *Qi*, ... fright confuses *Qi*, ... concentration focuses *Qi*, ..." (teachings from *Accepting Pain*, chapter 39 *Fengtong* 奉痛 of the *Huangdi Neijing, Suwen*).

"In conclusion, if people select the flavors of their food and mix them well, their skeleton will be straight, their muscles will have tone, their *Qi* and blood will circulate freely, their pores will be small and fine, therefore they will have reserves of *Essential Qi* and *Qi* in their bones. Follow this way and live a long life," advises *The Way Heaven Produces Qi*, chapter 3 *Shengqi Daotian* 生氣道天 in the *Huangdi Neijing, Suwen*.

Over two and a half millennia ago Chinese medical science developed a complex concept of bio-energy *(Qi)*. Currently, Western medical science is developing a complex concept of pain as expressed in a book published in +1996, *The Chronic Pain Control Workbook*:

> More recent theories have shown that the experience of pain is not a simple cause-and-effect relationship between the body and the brain. Rather, it is a complex web of pain signals, chemical messengers, emotions, and thoughts involving several different pathways of pain (page 15).

The Greatest Unsolved Mystery

The concepts of science include fact, theory and the unknown. Scientists develop theories to study the unknown and when possible, establish facts. In a few fields like mathematics and computer science, established facts and theory dominate the unknown. It is a fact that the unknown numeric value of pi (π) will remain unknown, because it is a number expressed by an infinite series of non-repeating digits. It is a fact computers never do what you **want**, they only do what you **command**. It is unknown why computers crash when you least expect it. Physics has a high fact/theory ratio, yet the unknown lies mostly beyond the reach of instruments. For example, inside the atom or deep in outer space. In geology the unknown lies deep within the Earth, such as, what mechanism drives the magnetic field and what process produces volcanic hot spots? In paleontology the reasons behind the great mass extinctions and the major ice ages are unknown. In archeology artifacts and theories guide the deciphering of unknown and unwritten chapters in human history.

In biology, new theories frequently replace old theories while biologists try to understand many complex unknown domains including cellular mechanics, biochemical reactions and genetic codes. While biologists have discovered many of the mechanisms of life, there remain many mysteries inside the human body and brain. "Cosmology has a reputation as a difficult science, but in many ways explaining the whole universe is easier than understanding a single-celled animal," wrote physicists Martin A. Bucher and David N. Spergel in their article "Inflation in a Low-Density Universe" in *Scientific American* magazine, January +1999.

Pain, out of sight and in the shadows, is chief among the many mysteries of the human body. Relief from pain has always been one of the main goals of medicine, yet there is very little agreement about pain—except that it hurts. Everyone knows pain when they feel it, but what they are feeling remains a mystery. Many ancient writers believed all disease was a divine punishment, as indicated by the original Latin meaning of pain as penalty or punishment. The Book of Job in the Bible represents pain as a test of faith.

The Stoics believed pain was good; Epicureans believed pain was bad. Aristotle taught that pain is an emotion like fear, anger and love. Hippocrates wrote that pain is a symptom of disease. Descartes reasoned that pain is a sensation like hot, cold and pressure; this is still the dominant scientific theory.

David B. Morris wrote in *The Culture of Pain*, "One crucial place to begin is with the acknowledgment that, despite our high-tech laboratories and surgical innovations, pain remains one of the most perplexing mysteries of our time. There is no authority today who can tell us exactly what pain is and how it works. Pain thus plunges us instantly into the midst of controversy and the unknown" (page 21).

Today, a growing number of doctors prefer to think of pain not as an external stimulation perceived by the brain's pain center (called a sensation), but as an individually interpreted physical-mental experience (called a perception), which includes mind and emotions. Changing the definition does not change the fact pain is a mystery. Today, a growing amount of scientific knowledge about the human body is available, yet an even deeper understanding of the biochemistry of injuries, the neuro-pathways in the brain and the at-

16

titudes of patients is needed. Pain is a bigger mystery than ever. Today, a growing number of drugs are available to treat suffering and yet the best way to relieve pain remains a mystery.

In ancient times in the West and throughout time in Eastern cultures, people reduced pain and promoted healing with touch. They developed theories about nature's healing power, an energy that is ignored by modern science. Why not use this mysterious *Qi* energy to heal your mysterious pain?

"The opposite of a correct statement is a false statement. But the opposite of a profound truth may well be another profound truth," said Professor Niels Bohr, the father of quantum physics and winner of the Nobel Prize for Physics in +1922.

Today, growing numbers of people are using the ancient science of acupuncture and acupressure with its concept of biological energy to treat their pain. Now you can make a quantum leap in your understanding of health and disease by studying the nature of pain in your own body. The best way to study energy is by learning to change pain into energy.

Pain Goes When Energy Flows

Pain (blocked energy) is like a friend who offers critical advice to save us from making mistakes. Some pain also helps locate energy to overcome difficult problems. This energy may be experienced during acupressure treatments. When this energy flows freely throughout the body, health is easily maintained. Health is like a fair-weather friend who cannot be found when things get rough or goes away when ignored.

Although you can feel this energy, it does not correspond to known scientific phenomena. Since you cannot see this energy it helps to visualize it as light and dark. Pain indicates either golden healing energy or dark disease energy. Golden energy with its glowing flowing feeling comes from pressure-sensitive pain points. Dark energy comes with chronic diseases which are thought of as deficient, stagnant, stuck and frozen energy. Dark disease energy opposes the golden healing energy.

Pressure on some painful places will release golden energy, but places with dark pain require healing energy released from elsewhere. Chronic pain that cannot be relieved by rubbing and pressing indicates dark energy, while pain that can be relieved by pressure is golden energy. This golden energy can then be used to relieve chronic pain and other symptoms as well as speed the healing of disease and increase the energy for living.

The Experience
of *Qi* Energy

Pain is blocked energy called injured *Qi*, whereas the feeling of energy flowing in the body is called *Got Qi (DEQI* 得氣 sounds like "duh chee"). It is defined as the experience of bodily sensations following the application of therapeutic pressure, acupuncture, or heat. The changing, moving sensations can feel like tingling, numbness, aching and soreness. After awhile a subtle, glowing, flowing feeling along the length of the body may be noticed.

If at first you do not feel energy sensations *(deqi)* when your acupoints are pressed, keep trying. It may be you need more practice at finding the points or it could be your *Qi* system has atrophied because of inactivity. The energy system will atrophy like other body systems when not used. Just as play and exercising keeps muscles strong, and reading and learning keeps the mind sharp, exercising your energy points allows you to feel stronger energy sensations. When you begin exercising after months of inactivity, muscles will complain and refuse to work. Then as you persist you become stronger until what was once difficult becomes easy. It takes knowledge and practice to develop skill. A Chinese proverb implores, "Bugs do not nest in a busy doorway."

Listen to your body as it talks about injured *Qi* (pain) while you look for *Qi* points to release golden energy. Locate known energy reserves and learn to free trapped energy. It is natural to hold, rub and press where it hurts. Pain will teach you all you need to know about your body's energy system. While learning, start with the easy pains that release golden energy. This takes about ten minutes. Listening to your body and locating energy points works best in a place where you will not be disturbed so you can relax as much as necessary.

If you have a sore or painful place on your arm or leg which is easy to reach, start there. Otherwise, start examining your neck and shoulders. Rub and press painful spots until you find that the pain subsides as you hold it. Rub and press gently at first. Slowly rub all around the most tender spot. Then focus on the most tender spot and press there. Press for about one minute. Press hard enough to feel the pain but not hard enough to cause tension in your body. Press into that gray area between pleasure and pain where the most energy can be released. The appropriate pressure will reduce the pain, which will release golden energy. It seems curious, but the best golden energy points are usually not very sore at all.

If at first you don't succeed try, try again. Keep exercising your energy system. If you are having trouble feeling energy, try using fewer stimulants and relaxants including painkillers, alcohol and coffee. They are numbing and result in the disruption of *Qi*.

Specific points on the body, called acupoints, will easily release golden energy for health and healing. Some of the most powerful points have been used since ancient times. An acupoint is usually the most tender spot in an area. These same acupoints become hypersensitive when corresponding parts of the body need help. However, it is interesting to note, even when acupoints are surprisingly hypersensitive with dark energy disease, you might not notice these points if you were not looking for them. This book describes in detail, twenty-eight acupressure acupoints that warn of disease and supply the body with golden energy.

Your Energy

This book introduces you to your energy system. Energy has been ignored by most of us and passed over by our doctors, but it is as much a part of us as our muscle, bone and brain. The secret to experiencing this energy system is revealed in this book. Experiencing the energy system is one of the many secrets discovered by ancient Chinese healers. Each point is different, which requires knowing the secret of that point. Read about and experience each point. There are hidden messages and pathways waiting for you to discover so you can change pain into energy. The way to find this energy is to explore your body for energy release points.

Be curious about energy spots and pain spots. Look for energy as if you were looking for gold. If you were to go on a treasure hunt for gold, you would need a map indicating where gold is likely to be found. You would also need to learn the signs the earth reveals to indicate where gold may be located. Gold is found in streambeds. As water erodes a mountain, gold is washed down and into streams, but not too far because it is so heavy. If the washout cuts into a vein of gold, it can be mined. For recovering gold you would also need supplies and tools. The only tools you will need to discover *Qi* energy are your hands. The map of energy points has been supplied by the ancient Chinese. This book explains how to use your hands as tools to discover where your body holds a treasure trove of golden energy.

The following exercise is designed to help you experience energy. First become aware of your energy state. Sit comfortably while answering these questions and fill in the chart to evaluate your energy system. Rate each body part for pain and energy aliveness. Sometime later you may want to evaluate each body part slowly—you may even take notes—but for now, take one minute or less. After some practice it will be as easy as reading the words in a book. As you read the body part ask yourself, "Is there pain or do I feel energy?"

Energy–Pain Chart

Scan the following body parts, while rating their energy-pain sensations: right foot, left foot, right leg, left leg, right

Energy–Pain Chart	Throb- bing Energy	Pulsing Energy	Tingly Energy	Numb- ness	Mild Pain	Uncom- fortable Pain	Distress- ing Pain	Feel Nothing
Right Foot								
Left Foot								
Right Leg								
Left Leg								
Right Hand								
Left Hand								
Right Arm								
Left Arm								
Abdo- men								
Chest								
But- tocks								
Back								
Neck								
Head								

hand, left hand, right arm, left arm, abdomen, chest, buttocks, back, neck and head. Copy the Energy–Pain Chart, and mark your answers to, "Is there pain or do I feel energy?" for each of the body parts.

If you have pain it's easier to experience energy. Pain

from a little injury makes the body stronger, whereas a great injury weakens the body. Chronic pain means the healing process has fatigued. Pain from a recent injury releases energy more easily than pain is released from chronic disease, but experienced energy workers find chronic pain just as easy to relieve though it may take more time. Some pain requires professional acupuncture, chiropractic or physical therapy treatments. Pain guides you to the hidden points, which release energy when pressed.

Pain is a message from your body that something is wrong. Your body needs help! You may have been told when something hurts, "Don't touch it," "Leave it alone" or "Ignore it. It'll go away." This way of thinking is not good for your health. Your body communicates in many ways. Pain communicates that your help is needed now and guides you to the points that will relieve the pain. **Touch your pain, feel your pain with your hands—not just your mind.** Rub and press when it feels good to do so, but stop what you are doing when it doesn't feel good. Don't aggravate your pain; get in touch with the place and the surrounding tissue. Rub for awhile. If it doesn't aggravate the pain, try pressing.

If rubbing aggravates the pain then stop rubbing. Find another nearby point that feels like it could release some energy. You may also find an acupoint listed in this book to rub and press. Look at the illustrated acupoint chart on page 200 for points nearest your pain. Try pressing several. Also, you may look in **Acupressure Therapy** on page 205 for suggested acupoints.

Rapid Healing

First lightly rub the area where it hurts, moving the skin around in circles or gently pressing and stroking. Then massage the area to feel the tissue. Look for tissue changes and patterns of pain. Finally, feel for the most painful points. Take your time, especially if the tissue feels hard and congested or if the pain is too intense. Make big circles to increase the circulation while you feel for other tender points. If it's tender, massage at that level of pressure. You may find lumps or bumps. Often you will feel painful rope-like muscles. It's common to find surprisingly painful places previously unknown to you.

After surveying the area, find the most painful point. Then press and hold it without moving. Relax and get comfortable. It may take time for your finger pressure to make a change. Hold the point and remain still until the pain changes. If it gets worse, lighten the pressure. If the pain gets better, keep holding while sensing the other changes. Does it feel tingly, heavy, less sharp or less sore? Do you feel something moving in your body? It may feel subtle. It may radiate a short or long distance. You may experience a tingly, glowing, flowing feeling. You may feel currents—some warm and some cold. Rubbing and pressing will remove the stagnant energy, which helps to restore proper circulation of blood and lymph. When you rub gently, stagnant energy is dispersed often resulting in the reduction of pain.

Most people don't experience energy sensations the first time they try, about half the people who try these methods will experience energy within minutes; a quarter will take days of practice. Some may never experience the energy sensations described in this book. A Chinese sage once said, "The journey of a thousand miles begins with the first step." The first time something new is tried, thoughts of failure, doubt and confusion sometimes surface. "What if I can't do it?" Not all people can feel *Qi*. It is a sense. Just as some people are color blind, some people can't feel energy sensations, even with the proper herbs and acupuncture.

Don't expect too much at first. Energy sensations are quieter than pain. Keep looking, massaging and exploring your body. Most everyone who explores the twenty-eight points described in this book will experience energy sensations at some of the acupoints.

24

Energy sensations are different than nerve sensations. Modern scientists in Japan and China have studied energy sensations extensively. In *Acupuncture: A Comprehensive Text* translated and edited by John O'Conner and Dan Bensky it states, "It was found that the perception of the conduction of the needle sensation was rather slow ..." (page 108). Nerve sensations are felt instantaneously. When you hit your elbow a certain way, your hand feels numb with "pins and needles." What has happened is a pinched nerve between the bones of the elbow caused the predictable sensation in the hand. The body feels normal elsewhere, except from the point where the nerve was pinched toward the extremity. This is a law that can be applied when locating nerve damage. It is said nerve damage is found between the altered sensation and the central nervous system.

When you provoke an energy sensation, the tingling feeling can travel toward the center of the body or toward the extremities. In contrast, when you hit a nerve, the instantaneous feeling is felt only in the direction of the extremity. Recall hitting your funny bone. In this way you can tell the difference between an energy sensation and a nerve sensation. Also, the energy sensation felt when pressing on a painful point or an acupressure point varies from one place to the next and from one person to another.

Change Disease into Health

Many Westerners define health as "not being sick." Health is the condition we enjoy when there is no disease. We think of health and disease as mutually exclusive. The ancient Far Eastern sages defined health as vitality and resilience when faced with life's challenges, or the ability to accept good and bad as part of life. We always have health and disease to some degree. Health is more than the absence of disease. Health is the ability to resist and recover from disease. It takes energy to be sick, just as it takes energy to play, dance, laugh or cry.

A cold is caused by a virus, according to Western medicine. A virus invades the body, and the immune system responds. We are wearing down our bodies because of the way we fight disease. A microorganism is identified, and a drug is used against it without consideration as to how the body will be affected by the invasion, or how the body will be affected by the drug. An ancient martial arts method suggests, "Gain information about and wear down the enemy by real and feigned attacks." What is important to Chinese medicine is how the body responds to invasion, rather than what caused the invasion.

The ancient Asians viewed medicine as the **art of prolonging life**. Thus, the mission of the ancient physician was **not** to treat the ill but to **guide** those who were not yet ill. In the second chapter of *The Yellow Sovereign's Classic*, the legendary physician, Qibo, explains this principle to the Yellow Sovereign, "To administer medicines for diseases already established and to suppress revolts already fomenting, is the same as people who begin digging a well after they have become thirsty, or like those who begin casting weapons after the battle has begun. Wouldn't these actions be too late?" This is the origin of the ancient saying, "A superior doctor treats when there is no disease."

Traditional Chinese medicine looks for how the body responds to the challenge of disease and assists the body in its task by making the body stronger.

Signs of Health

Most of us consider ourselves healthy, even though we may feel tired much of the time or have frequent nagging headaches or other pains that we treat with aspirin or other analgesics. Health is much more than the absence of disease. Consider these signs of health:

- Vitality, which is the energy you need to achieve what you want in your life. Vitality turns problems into challenges and everyday life into an adventure.

- A sense of humor, which enables you to take serious things lightly and light things seriously. It is the ability to laugh at yourself, to make friends out of enemies and to take a childlike joy in living.

- A good memory, which enables you to take advantage of present opportunities by remembering not only past victories and mistakes but also your dreams and goals for the future.

- The capacity to give freely, which means that you will continue to generate life. "The single grain hoarded produces nothing. Sown, it yields many times its number."

Symptoms of Disease

Western medicine seeks the cause of disease by identifying the pathogen that triggers the disease. Traditional Chinese medicine observes how the body responds to the pathogen. Western medicine then **attacks** the pathogen with drugs; traditional Chinese medicine **assists** the body in its fight against the pathogen.

Ancient Chinese sages refer to three great powers that influence each other: the Energy of Heaven, the Energy of Earth and Human Energy. The body changes in response to these three powers. The Energy of Heaven (天 Tian) is outside our skin and includes weather, climate and indoor environment. The Energy of Heaven (weather and sun) is transformed by the earth (biosphere). The Energy of Earth (地 Di) encompasses food and herbs, which affect the internal organs. Human (人 Ren) Energy includes thoughts and emotions changing in response to the energies of Heaven and Earth.

Disease occurs when the body adapts to unresolved stress or intense traumatic injury such as pollution, exposure, poor diet or intense emotion. Other causes include toxins, fatigue, injury and abuse of drugs and alcohol. Disease results when the body is actively healing itself or has given up healing, accepting and adjusting to the disease.

What is your relationship to pain and disease? Are pain and disease the enemy of health and happiness, or are they like true friends who help us for a short time but do not stay? Take your body in hand, place pressure on disease and change disease into health as the ancient Chinese did!

Ancient Asia

Acupressure is one of America's newest healing arts—and one of Asia's oldest. Mythic sage-kings, the very founders of Chinese culture, wrote books on acupuncture, massage, nutrition, divination (psychology), and herbs. The medical literature from ancient China is vast and wide. Countless numbers of medical books of all types have been published; hundreds are still available today.

The two oldest medical classics in use for over two millennia are *The Yellow Sovereign's Classic of Internal Medicine (Huangdi Neijing* 黃帝內經), hereafter referred to as *The Yellow Sovereign's Classic,* and *The Inspired Farmer's Classic of Herbal Pharmacopeia (Shennong Bencaojing* 神農本草經) hereafter referred to as *Shennong's Herbal.* A third book sometimes counted as a medical classic is the three-millennia-old *I Ching (Yijing* 易經 the *Classic of Change).*

Twenty-four centuries ago *The Yellow Sovereign's Classic,* a large medical compendium (first mentioned in historical documents around -400), advised doctors in China about relieving pain and curing disease. This book can be read today from several good English translations. Twenty-two centuries ago *Shennong's Herbal* (first mentioned in historical documents around -200) described the medicinal value of 365 herbs.

These ancient books were attributed to mythical sage-kings believed to have lived over two thousand years earlier. During the misty dawn of Chinese civilization the Three Sage-kings (三皇 Sanhuang sounds like "sahn who +wong") ruled the world. Their names were Fuxi (伏羲 sounds like "foo sheh"), Shennong (神農 sounds like "shen nong") and Huangdi (黄帝 sounds like "who+wong deh"). Notice that Sanhuang and Huangdi have the identical sound huang but have different characters and meanings. The former means "sage-king" and the latter means "yellow." It is common for different characters to have the same sound.

Where did these healing traditions come from? How was historical information preserved and transmitted? What evidence do we have for medicine in ancient China? To answer these questions let's scrutinize the remarkable and fascinating legends and myths traditionally believed by these organized, curious and intelligent people from the inscrutable Far East. Fortunately ancient Chinese history is easy to grasp because of the colorful persons involved. Scholars consider traditional dates before -800 (2,800 years ago) inaccurate and have adjusted the dates based on independent archeological data.

China's Ancient Rulers

Traditional Dates	From	To	Total Years
3 Sage-kings (Sanhuang)	-2852	-2575	277
5 Sovereigns (Wudi)	-2575	-2205	370
Xia dynasty	-2205	-1767	438
Shang dynasty	-1766	-1122	644
Zhou dynasty	-1122	-255	687
Warring States	-475	-221	254
Qin dynasty	-221	-207	14
Han dynasty	-206	+221	427

The ancient Chinese believed the future depended on their ancestors. They made offerings and prayed to their ancestors. The best things in life came from harmonious relations within the family. As Confucius said, "All men are brothers."

The Three Sage-kings mentioned above will be discussed later in this book.

The Five Sovereigns (五帝 Wudi sounds like "woo deh") were the legendary lords who ruled by birthright, important to clans as hereditary ancestors. Their names were often at the head of genealogies kept by royal families. They are often cited as models of ideal behavior for royalty, especially the primary king, the priest-king who held the title Son of Heaven. He prayed, performed rituals and offered animal sacrifices to the Lord Above, (also titled Heaven) who was the primary god. Lesser gods were also honored by the king. However, the ancient Chinese did not have a separate class of priests. There was a hierarchy in heaven just as there was on Earth.

The mythical Xia (夏 sounds like "she+ahh") dynasty was founded by the Great Yu, who used earthworks to change the course of the Yellow River and drained flooded land making it safer for farmers. The dynasty is believed to have reigned for over four centuries farming the ancient Yellow River Basin.

All information on the Xia ruling clan is received from the archives of succeeding dynasties and published in China's three ancient classics, the *Classic of (Historical) Documents* (書經 *Shujing)*, the *Classic of Songs* (詩經 *Shijing)* and the most comprehensive Han dynasty (-200) history book, *Records of the Historian* (史記 *Shiji)*. China's most ancient classic is the *Classic of Documents (Shujing),* a few of which are said to have originated during the Xia dynasty. No independent written records have been unearthed to date. In fact, no archeological find has shed light on the Xia ruling clan, but tradition says they ruled over forty-two centuries ago.

The legendary Shang (商 sounds like "Shang" as in Shanghi) dynasty was founded by a warrior king who defeated the last corrupt Xia ruler over thirty-seven centuries ago (traditional date) with a superior army of chariots. Thus the Mandate of Heaven changed to acknowledge the Shang king as priest and Son of Heaven. The nobles drove classy sports carts and the army used war chariots. The ancient Shang made beautiful bronze ceremonial vessels prized by today's collectors and museums. They farmed the rich loam basin for over six centuries and became incredibly wealthy. The last Shang capitol was built after the Yellow River changed its course. The site of the new capitol, called Yin, was built at today's Anyang near the middle of the Yellow River basin. It soon became the largest city in the world. Wealth and power caused the kings to become decadent and cruel. The last Shang dynasty's king outraged everyone with his inhumane treatment of respected rulers. He imprisoned an innocent prince who would someday be called King Wen.

The legendary sage, King Wen (文王 Wen Wang sounds like "when Wang") was a child prodigy as a prince of the Zhou (周 sounds like "Joe") clan. While the Shang clan was the center of Chinese culture, the Zhou clan farmed and ranched in the wild west, surrounded by barbarians. The Zhou clan's ruling family was given a well-rounded education as scholars. King Wen built up a prosperous state in the Wei River valley west of the decadent Shang dynasty. His eldest son defeated the Shang king's army in one decisive battle, and because of his wise strategies very few lives were lost. King Wen and another son, the Duke of Zhou, wrote the *I Ching* (易經 *Yijing* sounds like "E ching" the *Classic of Change)*, a divination handbook. Therefore, King Wen was a scholar priest-king. The *I Ching* has been published continuously since the time of Confucius (b. -551, d. -479), who may have edited it and added eight of ten commentaries to the sixty-four hexagrams developed by the sage King Wen.

The Zhou dynasty built its first capital city in the Wei River valley, west of the Yellow River basin over three millennia ago (traditional date -1122, adjusted -1050 to -1025). The problem of ruling such a large area was solved by establishing two capitals. They kept their mountain homeland in the west as the primary capital and established a secondary capital in the east. The descendants of King Wen ruled wisely for three centuries from the Western Zhou homeland.

When the Zhou dynasty's western capital was destroyed by barbarians (-771), the king moved east and built a new capital near the old secondary capital. Three hundred years later China deteriorated into the Warring States period (-475 to -212), when the weak and corrupt Eastern Zhou rulers, surrounded by many strong states, tried to act as mediator. Without power, little could be done. For two hundred and fifty years stronger states took advantage of weaker states because they didn't fear the feeble Zhou dynasty. They lost faith in the Son of Heaven but did not covet the office. Chaos prevailed and crime increased, while the morals of ruling families deteriorated. Many philosophies vied for the attention of the kings and royal leaders of the warring clans. At the same time, the two aforementioned medical classics emerged.

The Qin (秦 sounds like "cheen") king cunningly conquered the clans in the Wei River valley west of the warring states in the Yellow River basin. He went on to ruthlessly defeat the warring kings and founded the Qin dynasty over twenty-two hundred years ago. Therefore, he was said to be cunning and ruthless like a tiger. The First Emperor (始皇帝 Shi Huangdi sounds like "sure who+wong deh") ruled over a united empire nearly the size of China today. He's the guy everybody loves to hate because he burned all the books he didn't like and buried many scholars alive. The First Emperor died in -210 after ruling only eleven years and his son ascended the throne. The Qin dynasty reigned for a mere fifteen years. Archeologists have since unearthed an army of "larger than life" terra cotta soldiers guarding his tomb.

In the meantime, a rebel commoner from the Han (漢 sounds like "hahn") clan fought and won many difficult battles and rose to the rank of general. As a general he built alliances with other strong states that opposed the cruel king of Qin. He led the allies to victory over the infamous Qin dynasty. The peasant general became the Han dynasty's first emperor; his clan's dynasty reigned for four centuries.

The two medical classics, *The Yellow Sovereign's Classic* and *Shennong's Herbal* emerged in China at about the same time books attributed to Hippocrates (traditional date b. -460, d. -377), a Greek physician who is regarded as the Father of Western Medicine, were written. Some thirty years later Alexander the Great (b -356, d. -323) inherited the kingdom of Macedonia, a barely civilized state west of Greece. He conquered the Western world from Greece to India and from Persia to Egypt. Tragically, he died before consolidating control over his empire. His generals became governors who fragmented the empire, establishing control in conquered areas. These warring states fought each other until Rome established the Pax Romana about three hundred years later. He did not live to see it, but the Greek (Hellenic) culture has had a lasting influence throughout the Western world.

Medical Mystery Proves Myth to be History

The mythical Three Sage-kings of antiquity are considered an invention of people trying to reconstruct their heritage by claiming to be related to heroic founders of their culture. The ancient medical books, *The Yellow Sovereign's Classic* and *Shennong's Herbal* were written by unknown authors twenty-four hundred years ago (-400) and attributed the writing to these ancient sage-kings. The claim that the Shang (from -1766 to -1122) and early Zhou dynasty (from -1122 to -771) each reigned for over five hundred years in peace and harmony has been classified alongside folktales as pure myth. The short biographies of these mythical Chinese Three Sage-kings (Sanhuang) describe them as talented human beings acting in remarkable but ordinary ways rather than acting supernaturally.

Western myths such as the Sumerian *Gilgamesh,* the *Iliad* and the *Odyssey* of the Greeks and the Hindu *Mahabharata* and *Ramayana* are lengthy epics involving supernatural persons acting in ways full of imagery, but obviously fanciful. Ancient Chinese culture has nothing to compare. Instead, ancient Chinese classics are either short poems or historical clan records. The poems were actually songs performed in traditional choreographed dance, accompanied by music. These songs were composed to entertain and communicate ideas.

During a time when traditions were being forgotten by a decadent society, Confucius and his disciples kept them alive. They gathered frequently to beat drums, sing songs and dance. Confucius gleaned over 300 short poems from clan libraries and compiled a songbook of greatest hits called *The Classic of Songs (Shijing).*

Most of these songs have a moral message on topics including: temple rituals, love sickness, the joys of courtship, wedding ceremonies, married life, tragic separations, lost love, child birthing and rearing, faithful children, dutiful officials, virtuous ancestors, the misery of famine, the difficulties of war, martial victories and memorable deeds.

Clan records reflect scrupulous interest in honoring ancestors by remembering them. From ancient times (and to some extent to this day) the presence of dead ancestors was as real as the existence of the living. Ancestors ruled the world of the living and the living were expected to remember and pay respect or suffer the consequences. Ancestors could help or hurt the living by revealing the Will of Heaven or by bringing good weather and good health, but if forgotten, they brought catastrophic weather and disease. Ancestral lineage is important to this day, as a trip to San Francisco's Chinatown reveals when a public ancestral temple is visited.

From ancient times clans kept two sets of records: lineage tablets and tablets for recording significant events and speeches important to members of the clan. Even when a clan was defeated in war, out of fear of retribution from the ancestors of the vanquished, the tablets were preserved in a separate library by an archivist. History records the name of one such man who compiled a book of wisdom. His name is given as Lao Tzu (traditional date b. -604). The importance of preserving the knowledge of the ancestors out of fear of retribution has one exception: First Emperor Qin Shi Huang-di, who burned all the archives. Whether he was fearless in defying tradition or was fearful that the past would over-shadow him is not known.

From as far back in time as the Zhou dynasty, there were four classes of people: royalty/ennobled, scholar/warrior, peasant/farmer and merchants (the lowest class in ancient China). Scholars and warriors descended from any class, however choosing to be a scholar or warrior was the only way for an upwardly mobile commoner to ascend to the circles of power. Scholars (士 shi sounds like "sure") were classically educated men employed as scribes, teachers, as-tronomers, astrologers, librarians and historians. Clans em-ployed the shi (scholars) as scribes to keep records and maintain the libraries of their ancestors. Large clans had professional historians. The ruling clan of the empire had a department headed by a Grand Historian (太士 Taishi sounds like "tie sure") staffed by many historians and scribes. They had the added responsibility of observing and recording astronomical events in order to correct and pub-lish an accurate imperial calendar (almanac) every year.

The shi (scholars) were an independent proud profession who recorded the day-to-day activities of royalty and impor-tant state events, including the good and bad deeds of the ruling elite. From prehistoric times, the department of as-tronomer and calendar maker was essential to the king, the Son of Heaven. These astronomers kept records of omens in the sky. They stayed up in shifts so as not to miss any signs in the heavens. Without this information they believed the king could lose the Mandate of Heaven, for if he failed to predict eclipses, natural disasters and planet locations, his failure would indicate a poorly run government.

The almanac was published and distributed to kings throughout the empire to predict the spring and autumn equinoxes and the winter and summer solstices as well as the location of planets in the sky. The Chinese Son of Heaven also established his authority over his subjects, an agricultural people, by publishing an Imperial calendar every year, which was a true *Farmers Almanac* given to clans in exchange for tribute and allegiance. The almanac included advice on planting, cultivating and harvesting, animal husbandry, raising silk worms and making silk.

During the Zhou dynasty an 'outer' records office for non-clan records was established with a separate librarian. Included in the library were books about farming, the *Eight Trigrams* (八卦 *Bagua* sounds like "ba goo+ah"), official histories of other clans such as *The Three Sage-kings* (三皇 *Sanhuang*) and *The Five Sovereigns (Wudi)*. Confucius visited these libraries and used his knowledge of ancient scripts to popularize ancient songs and his clan's history and ethics. It is said Confucius visited Lao Tzu, who was such a librarian.

The earliest and foremost philosophers, Confucius (b. -551, d. -479) and Mencius (b. -372, d. -289), wrote about non-religious humanistic ideals. Many other books on philosophy followed, such as the mystical writings of Lao Tzu, the humorous Taoist writings in Chuang Tzu's (b. -369, d. -286) *The Classic of the Way* (道德經 *Daodejing* or *Tao Te Ching*) and the medical writings attributed to Huangdi, *The Yellow Sovereign's Classic of Internal Medicine*. Many books advised the king on military strategies, such as the martial writings of Sun Tzu's (b. -298, d. -238) *The Art of War*. Many western readers are familiar with these books.

A Medical Mystery

In the year 1899, in the city of Beijing, a writer named Liu Tieyun (sounds like "Lee+you tie UN") suffered from malaria. Mr. Liu went to a local herb pharmacy and purchased traditional Chinese herbs for treating malaria. For over three thousand years medicinal soups have been simmered in a particular way to extract the medicinal properties of herbs. Traditional Chinese herbs for treating malaria included roots, twigs, berries and 'dragon bone,' a fossil bone used in medicine that cools inflammation. In his bag of herbs, he was shocked to find a strange writing on the dragon bone. He recognized it as more primitive but similar to the written glyphs found on Shang bronze vessels prized by collectors.

Mr. Liu acquired more dragon bones with ancient writings and began to study them, discussing his findings with archeologists. After some detective work, they discovered that the bones came from the center of the Yellow River basin's Anyang district (location of the mythical kingdom of Shang) in Henan. Farmers found thousands of fossil turtle shells and shoulder blades from cattle and deer while plowing their fields and had sold them to local druggists. Herbalists have been using fossil bones (a source of minerals) for thousands of years. Some of these bones actually come from dinosaurs believed to be the remnants of dragons, therefore the name 'dragon bones.' These mysterious writings on medicinal dragon bones were a key to unlocking the ancient language of China. Dragon bones with Shang writing on them became known as Shang Oracle Bones.

During the early twentieth century, historians were skeptical of all books and historical dates prior to the burning of the books by Qin Shi Huangdi. Much of traditional history is found in the *Records of the Historian (Shiji),* written about one hundred years later. With the advent of modern scientific skepticism, scholars believed the succeeding Han dynasty, founded by a commoner, must have ordered its grand historian to make up a lineage beginning with the Yellow Sovereign. They reasoned that since all the books had been burned, he was free to use folk stories and fabrications.

Sima Qian (sounds like "see ma chee+ahn"), who was born sixty years after the founding of the Han dynasty, authored the *Records of the Historian,* a history of the defeat of the Qin dynasty and the founding of the Han Empire. It included historical information on the Xia, Shang and Zhou Dynasties. He was suspected by early twentieth century scholars of having fabricated sections of the histories prior to the infamous burning of the books.

Records of the Historian

Sima Qian (b. -145, d. -90) wrote the *Records of the Historian (史記 Shiji),* China's first comprehensive history book. It reports on people and events from the founding of the Han dynasty (漢朝) back to ancient times. His history included minorities and foreign countries, eight essays on ritual, music, law, calendars, astronomy, sacrifice, water control and weights and measures, king lists from twelve clans, ten tables of historical events and many detailed biographies of kings, princes, generals, ministers, scholars, doctors, merchants, assassins and diviners. He attempted to separate fact from legend and in so doing wrote a history of the known world.

This project was initiated by his father Sima Tan, Grand Historian of the Han clan. While his father dreamed of a comprehensive history, and gathered material at the Han capital, the younger Qian traveled widely, verifying information in the clan archives and collecting and researching historical information. At thirty-two he succeeded his father as grand historian. In honor of his father's dying request, Qian continued writing the history when he was forty-two. After seven years of labor on the manuscript, tragedy interrupted his work.

China was again defending the border from the northern Hun barbarians. Emperor Wu wanted the leader of the Huns captured or at least forced to recognize the authority of the Han dynasty. He dispatched several armies numbering thousands of men, but to no avail. One such army, led by the brave General Li Ling (sounds like "Lee ling"), after initial success against the barbarians, tried a daring raid deep into Hun territory. Though outnumbered, he marched into the heart of the enemy camp with several thousand infantrymen shouting taunting challenges at the Hun chief. For ten days he engaged the enemy in combat, but the Huns received support from distant warlords. Every man, woman and child summoned came to the defense of the great Hun chief. Realizing his rouse had failed, General Li retreated south. For thousands of miles his men fought until all their arrows were exhausted and the road was blocked. Relief forces did not come to help them escape.

General Li's army fought to the death, but he was captured. When Emperor Wu heard General Li had been captured he became angry and defamed his name. All the court officials agreed with the emperor and discredited the general's efforts with the exception of Sima Qian. He had known General Li and believed him to be one of the finest men of his time, so he recounted the general's heroic deeds. For this impertinence he was arrested, imprisoned and tortured. Finally the emperor decided to inflict the most disgraceful punishment of castration. An aristocrat would often commit suicide rather than be subjected to this humiliation, but Qian had not completed the manuscript he had promised his father, Sima Tan. So "dwelling in vileness and disgrace" he completed the history when he was fifty years old.

Sima Qian claimed to be a skeptical meticulous historian. He further claimed to have access to carefully preserved clan histories that survived the book burning. He states in his book that he omitted what he could not verify from two or more sources. He included critical comments about the source material available to him. He was meticulous about accuracy and attended to detail as is required of his profession.

Sima Qian changed the way history was written. He wrote an interesting history that was easy to read in a popular style. It became the standard for historians throughout Asia. Appended at the end of chapters are his acute critical comments about his sources.

Sima Qian consulted archives that had been maintained for thousands of years. However, he knew nothing of the Shang Oracle Bones. Today, we have two independent sources of information on the Shang dynasty, the oracle bones of Shang and the historical records of Sima Qian. Modern historians have compared these records and have found Sima Qian's errors to be as he said, errors of omission.

Kings regularly changed the way calendars were made since the Yellow Sovereign (*Huangdi*) invented calendar making. Because of many changes to the calendars used for the last thousand years, the years varied when calculating backwards, therefore dates became inaccurate the farther back in time Qian went. When in doubt, he omitted dates. Nonetheless, his dates were found to be accurate after -800.

Notes from Shang Dynasty Oracle Bones

When the dragon bones used in medicine to solve health problems were discovered to have ancient Shang writing used in divination, the name Shang Oracle Bones originated. The Shang culture was based on farming and ranching. They employed advanced technology in making large intricate bronze vessels and fine silk. They had horses, chariots and a writing system.

Because Shang shamans wrote notes on bones about their divination concerns, we are now learning about life in ancient China over three millennia ago. Topics covered include weather forecasts, crop reports, best travel times, war strategies, hunting reports and health problems. The divination process is unknown. All that remains of the ritual are the oracle bones.

The Shang priest-kings had a reciprocal relationship with the Supreme Sovereign Shangdi (sounds like "shang deh; deh as in duck"; shang means "above" or "supreme" and di means an "hereditary ancestor" or "Sovereign"). The priest-king was the Son of Heaven and therefore the only intermediary who could intervene between all humans and the Lord Above (Supreme Sovereign). The Shang king's shaman also used the bones to consult and appease the lineage ancestors of the Shang.

Modern scholars analyzing the patterns of marks left as a result of the oracle bone divination process have discovered similarities to the patterns inherent in the *I Ching* (易經 *Classic of Change)*. The divination notes also mention Shang kings and other historical events commented upon in the *I Ching*. The Duke of Zhou finished the book his father, King Wen, began writing while wrongfully imprisoned for seven years. These priest-king scholars used the same divination system as the Shang priest-kings, but codified it into the diviner's promptbook we now know as the *I Ching*.

By 1952 modern scholars had collected 161,989 pieces of oracle bones unearthed at Anyang. Many more caches from the Shang and Zhou dynasties have been unearthed since. The writing consists of forty-five hundred characters with approximately seventeen hundred of the most common glyphs having been deciphered. The glyph for disease is the image of an ill person lying in bed at home 疒. Thirty-six distinct diseases have been noted on the bones.

The diseased appeased the deceased with prayers, gifts and animal sacrifices; when all of these failed to heal them, they resorted to exorcism. There is no mention of acupuncture or herbs. However, in the Shang digs, stones used in acupuncture and medicinal herbs were unearthed. Just because the oracle bones indicate divination was used, it does not indicate that other therapeutic methods were not used to aid in the cure of diseases. It would be surprising, even suspect, if these scraps of divination notes described anything other than the Shang king's concerns communicated to Shangdi and the deceased.

The Shang astronomer-diviners used a ten-day week and a double month of sixty days with each day having a unique name composed of two characters. They calculated with numbers using a base ten place-value notation. This is identical to the system we use today and not the primitive roman numerals, which make it difficult to multiply and divide. They observed a calendar year of 365.25 days (actually 365.242-199) and a lunation cycle of 29.53 days (actually 29.530-588). They used a gnomon to adjust the calendar. A gnomon is an upright stick or standing stone used as a natural clock and calendar. It acts as a sundial measuring the time of day as the shadow moves from west to east. It can be used to determine the time of year by measuring the length of the noon shadow as it changes from long in the winter to short in the summer.

The knowledge obtained from the notes on the oracle bones verified the correctness of Sima Qian's ancient historical writings earlier questioned by skeptical scientists. They also shed light on historical Shang kings briefly mentioned in other classics such as the *Classic of Documents* and the *Classic of Songs* selected by Confucius. Further study enabled modern historians and scientists to determine the dates individual kings reigned, because the records included the dates when eclipses of the moon and sun occurred. Six lunar eclipses were identified (-1361, -1342, -1328, -1311, -1304, -1217) and one solar eclipse (-1217) plus many meteor showers. The Shang divination scholars noted the earliest record of a star gone nova twenty-three hundred years ago (-1300). One such note translates, "On the seventh day of the month, a great new star appeared in company with

Antares." Many days later it was written, "the new star dwindled."

Examination of additional divination notes reveal King Wuding (-1324, mentioned in the historical records) suffered from eye problems; his son had headaches; and it was a bad sign that Hao (sounds like "how"), a pregnant consort's baby, was presenting breech, and she could die. Also, King Chen had tooth decay and stomachaches; many concubines complained of gynecological disorders.

Records of Ancient Astronomers

Chinese records from all sources of astronomical and meteorological observations are continuous and accurate from -500 and are a faithful record of celestial events for three thousand years (starting about -1300). Today's archeologists and anthropologists have available records of uncertain dates going back to -2000. Chinese records are the only astronomical records for thousands of years before the European Middle Ages, around the year 1000.

In Neolithic times (-3700 to -2000) the Chinese used sighting tubes for observing the heavens. Chinese historical books record the appearance of many comets. The recording of so many comets is unprecedented in history. Scientists have computed the orbits of forty comets before the year 1500 using Chinese records almost entirely.

The evidence of the Shang Oracle Bones corroborates traditional notions of the Shang dynasty. The dates of kings have been adjusted and we have more detailed information concerning their individual lives than would be necessary to prove a case in court. So the medicinal dragon bones with mysterious writing prove the once-thought-mythical Shang dynasty is truly history.

Three Sage-kings of Antiquity

The Three Sage-kings (三皇 Sanhuang) are the mythical founders of Chinese civilization. They could be thought to represent three traditions in prehistoric society. A clan from the **east,** represented by the color **green,** had a tradition of taming animals as nomadic herders and used a system of classification called the Eight Trigrams. A clan from the **south,** represented by the color **red,** had a tradition of farming (rice cultivation began in the south) and herb lore. A clan in the **middle**, represented by the color **yellow,** had a tradition of civilization incorporating, from all directions, the best of everything including medicine.

Animal Tamer (Fuxi 伏羲 sounds like "foo sheh" traditional date of his reign -2852), the Father of Chinese Philosophy, is first of the Three Sage-kings. He was the leader of a nomadic group who settled and ranched cattle and sheep. He invented pictographs called wen (文 sounds like "when"), *Yinyang* (陰陽 sounds like "y+een yah+ng ") philosophy and the Eight Trigrams (八卦 *Bagua* sounds like "ba goo+ah") classification system, later developed by King Wen (文王 Wen Wang translates as Culture King or Word King) and the Duke of Zhou (sounds like "Joe") now called the *I Ching* (*Yijing* 易經 sounds like "E ching" the *Classic of Change*). See the Bagua, page 59.

Confucius wrote a biography of Fuxi in his addendum called *Grand Commentary* to the *I Ching*. In antiquity Fuxi "ruled the world below heaven, looking up, he saw signs in Heaven (stars, weather), looking down, he saw methods on Earth (laws of nature). He talked to (cultured 文 wen) the birds and beasts. His body sensed all that is near and he sensed the distant (world) through signs. The Eight Trigrams are a good place to start, use its virtues to reach illuminating insights; use its categories to group innumerable things. He made knotted cords (used in record keeping) and snare nets for use in the field (to capture and tame animals) and in fishing."

Sima Qian was not confident Fuxi was historical, so he did not include him in the biography section of the *Records of the Historian*. See **Fuxi's Biography by Confucius** on page 232.

Inspired Farmer (神農 Shennong sounds like "shen nong" traditional date of his reign began -2752), the Father of Chinese Herbalists, is second of the Three Sage-kings. The first herb book known to be published is *Shennong's Herbal* (神農本草經). Sima Qian also left Shennong out of the biographies because he was not confident that Shennong was a historical figure. Sima Qian only recorded that Shennong tasted various herbs to discover their healing benefits and medicinal value and also that he discovered antidotes for poisonous plants.

Yellow Sovereign (Huangdi 黃帝 sounds like "who+ wong deh" traditional date b. -2674, d. -2575), is the Father of Chinese Civilization and third of the Three Sage-kings. The first Chinese medical compendium has been attributed to him and is called *The Yellow Sovereign's Classic* (黃帝 內經). Sima Qian had enough confidence in the records about Huangdi that he included his biography in the section about ancient kings. He may be the legendary figure who invented the first calendar. His calendar used cycles of 60 days, 60 moons and 60 years. The cycle system uses yin-yang and the five elements. He is said to have invented clothing, construction, coinage, bows and arrows, astronomy, music, and a writing system.

Traditionally, one or more posthumous titles were given to famous kings. This makes it difficult to be sure of the existence of Fuxi and Shennong as individuals. However, modern anthropologists would agree that the attributes of these individuals characterize the emergence of thought, socialization and civilization in ancient China.

The First Emperor

During the Warring States period (-475 to -212) the weak and corrupt Zhou ruler consolidated his capital in the Yellow River basin after the dynasty lost control of their capital and homeland in the Wei River valley to the west. At that time, the Wei River valley was ruled by the less civilized Qin clan, a small state that gradually gained power and absorbed a few local states. Further west of the Qin clan were primitive non-Chinese people. The Tocharian barbarians lived to the north-west in a high desert called the Tarim Basin. The Tibetans lived to the southwest in the Himalaya Mountains. To the east, in the great basin of the Yellow River, the remnants of the Zhou dynasty reigned.

The Qin dreamed of a time when a warrior king from their clan would graze horses beside the Yellow River. In time a young Qin prince of thirteen was groomed by the Legalist Prime Minister Li Si (sounds like "Lee zeh") to be a fierce leader. The philosophy of the Legalists advised that in order to gain power, a ruler should deceive, bribe and terrify the other states. While other philosophies encouraged ethical behavior, the Legalists suggested ignoring ethics and diplomacy. Ultimately they taught "might makes right." They further advocated strict controls and dire consequences for any violation of the law. When the Qin prince became King of Qin, he centralized power by encouraging agriculture and military strength and discouraged subversive activities such as art, poetry and philosophy.

In -212, by ruthlessly defeating the other warring states one after another, the Qin king became emperor of China, one hundred and eleven years after Alexander conquered the Western world. The once dreamed of future-warrior king extended the Qin clan's eastern borders to the Yellow River and beyond to the eastern sea (Korea), to the South China Sea (Vietnam), to the northern range of mountains which make a natural boundary to the Gobi Desert and to the Himalaya Mountains in the west.

In order to rule the Qin dynasty's vast empire, the Qin emperor established a rigid law and order government. To control the surviving royal families, he forcibly moved them to a luxurious new city in the Wei River valley. He tore down the walls surrounding all cities and divided the empire into thirty-six provinces administered by appointed governors. To efficiently manage the empire, he reformed the currency, re-distributed the land and taxed the farmers, who also sup-plied yearly labor.

The Qin emperor also standardized writing, weights and measures and the track width of wheels to fit a uniform width of highways. Mountainsides were leveled and valleys were filled to build straight, tree-lined, multi-laned highways with one lane reserved for the emperor's private use. The high-ways were supplemented by dredging rivers and digging in-terconnecting canal waterways for transportation of goods. This interstate transportation system extended throughout the empire. His captive soldiers and conscripts also built ex-tensive palaces and completed the Great Wall.

In the first year of his reign as the Son of Heaven, the king of Qin asked his scholars to suggest an imperial title acknowledging that instead of being a king among kings, he was now "the one and only ruler of the black haired people." His scholars suggested this had not been the case since the dawn of Chinese civilization, when the Five Di (五帝 Sover-eigns) and Three Huang (三皇 Sage-kings) ruled, and that their domain was small in comparison. The Qin king com-bined "Huang" with "Di" to create the title Huangdi (皇帝 "Sage King Sovereign" usually translated as Emperor). He decreed Huangdi would be used by his children for ten thou-sand generations. To distinguish his reign as the first, he added Shi (始 sounds like "sure"), which means beginning. His title then became Qin Shi Huangdi (秦始皇帝 Qin's First Emperor). Huangdi became the title assumed by em-perors of subsequent dynasties until modern times. For the next 2,100 years the Chinese empire had the basic bound-aries and bureaucratic administrative system he established.

In the eighth year of Qin Shi Huangdi's reign as the Son of Heaven, he sent unjust lawyers to work on the Great Wall. While holding a wine party for seventy scholars to wish him-

48

self long life, his archery captain toasted his keen mind, sage-like wisdom and great generosity. He congratulated the emperor for establishing peace across China with his unequaled military strength, allowing people to finally rest from hundreds of years of war and to find happiness. The First Emperor was very pleased until a Confucian scholar from Qi remarked that the Shang and Zhou dynasties ruled for about one thousand years with the traditional policy of sending sons, brothers or trusted officials to live with allied royal clans. The scholar suggested the policy of keeping clan royals in one city was unheard of since antiquity. He warned, "Your archery captain only flatters you. That could lead to errors in thinking. Be careful, he's not a loyal subject."

Li Si, who advised the emperor regarding Legalist policies, was now the chancellor. He replied that times had changed; the new empire was planned to last ten thousand generations. Li Si scoffed that it may be too difficult for a stupid Confucian scholar to understand; such scholars just stirred up trouble and disturbed the peace. He then lectured on the successes of the Legalist government and how the scholars who criticized the laws and proclamations ought to be eliminated. An ancient Chinese saying declares, "The tongue is a terrifying weapon; it destroys lives."

Chancellor Li Si went on to suggest prohibiting dissident speech and requested all historical records other than the Qin clan's be burned. Only officials allowed to posses them would be exempt. He wanted the *Classic of Songs* (詩經 *shijing*) and the *Classic of Documents* (書經 *shujing*) destroyed, as well as all books on other philosophies.

Acting on Li Si's advice, the First Emperor buried scholars alive and burned all books except practical ones on divination, forestry, agriculture and medicine. The Qin dynasty consisted of just two emperors, Qin Shi Huangdi and his son. The length of time the Qin family ruled was the shortest in China's four thousand year recorded history. The people grew weary of the oppressive policies of the Legalists and brought down the dynasty. It lasted only fifteen years.

The English word for China is believed to have its origin in the name of the Qin (Ch'in sounds like "cheen") dynasty; of course the Chinese people never used this term to refer to their country or its people. The Chinese term for China is Middle Kingdom (中國 Zhongguo). China is a land of many nationalities; however, the majority of ruling families have come from the Han nationality.

How fortunate that the First Emperor did not burn the medical writings of Huangdi. It is interesting that he created the title emperor (Huangdi 皇帝) with a different character sounding identical to the Yellow Sovereign (Huangdi 黃帝). The significance of this ploy is not lost on the Chinese ear. How ironic that the emperor who caused so much unnecessary pain saved a book *(The Yellow Sovereign's Classic)* that reveals the secret to the Chinese method of relieving pain.

Traditional Chinese Medicine

The healing arts of Asia apply principles attributed to the mythical Yellow Sovereign (traditional date b. -2697, d. -2597) which are found in *The Yellow Sovereign's Classic of Internal Medicine (Huangdi Neijing 黃帝内經)*. It is the oldest and only medical book in the world that has **never** gone out of print. It has guided the practice of Asian medicine for more than twenty-four hundred years. It describes how the forces of Heaven (天) and Earth (地) affect human (人) life and how people can stay healthy. Theories discussed include the causes of disease, the circulation of *Blood (XUE 血* sounds like "shoe+way"), the principle of *Yinyang* (陰陽 sounds like "y+een yah+ng") and the *Five Elements* (五行), which are symbolic states of change: water (水), wood (木), fire (火), earth (土) and metal (金). Unique medical methods are described including how to: feel the *Pulse (MAI 脈* sounds like "my"), analyze the symptoms, diagnose the constitution, and treat disease—methods still used today by doctors of Oriental medicine. Around the world today health practitioners use this knowledge in time-honored therapies including acupuncture, massage, herbology, nutrition and exercise.

In *The Yellow Sovereign's Classic* many far-sighted observations of nature and medical discoveries are evident. For instance, a description of the water cycle reveals that water vapor rises to form clouds; in clouds, water vapor condenses to form rain. (See **The Yellow Sovereign on the Cause of Pain** on page 238 for the text.) It describes biological cycles, which affect behavior and are disrupted by disease. Today, circadian rhythms evident in many plants and animals are studied by scientists. These internal clocks regulate hormone and organ functions.

The Yellow Sovereign's Classic was the first medical book to describe the circulation of blood through vessels pumped by the heart. Most science books attribute William Harvey with that discovery two millennia later in 1628. *The Yellow Sovereign's Classic* also goes into great detail about the importance of a balanced diet. Not only does it mention the importance of grains, vegetables and a little meat in a balanced diet, it also warns of imbalances caused by excessive consumption of certain foods. It observed excessive alcohol consumption results in a deficiency disease. An excess of rich food causes a thirsting and wasting disease we now know as diabetes. Diabetics have a deficiency of insulin. Today in the United States improved nutrition has eliminated serious deficiency diseases, with the exception of vitamin B deficiency which plagues alcoholics.

In *The Yellow Sovereign's Classic,* there are compiled the teachings of ancient healing masters regarding acupressure and acupuncture, as well as other Asian healing arts. These sages theorized that people receive energy from the air they breathe and from the food they eat. Mental and physical activity consumes this energy. Energy coordinates the interaction of body, mind and spirit. This energy also heals. However, healing depletes the body of *Qi* energy. When there are no blockages in the flow of *Qi* energy through the channels and crossings, and if one eats fresh food and breathes fresh air, then one experiences glowing health.

Disease can still affect an individual even though they are eating and breathing properly. Symptoms occur when the flow of *Qi* energy stagnates or the blood congeals, blocking the channels and crossings.

Symptoms of Injured *Qi*

- Physical pain
- Disability
- Mental confusion
- Emotional anxiety
- Depression
- Lack of energy to adequately perform tasks

Traditional Chinese medicine is a term used to describe Asian healing arts, which flourished throughout the Far East. During the reign of the First Emperor, Chinese medicine spread to Korea and Vietnam. Each culture adapted it to its own needs and temperament.

The Japanese, Koreans, Tibetans and Vietnamese developed indigenous forms of acupuncture, massage and herbology. Just as in China, many different traditions developed over several millennia, so it would be better to use the term "traditions" in Chinese medicine. The Chinese refer to biological energy as *Qi,* believing it flows through the body along channels called *meridians* (*JING* 經 sounds like "jeeng"). The Japanese written word *KI* is pronounced "key," while the Koreans say "gee." These all refer to the life force and all use the same character for *Qi* (氣).

The ancient Chinese healing masters discovered that reflex points on the *meridians* become sore when disease afflicts the body. Today acupressure therapists stimulate these points to move the flow of energy in the body, which restores proper functioning.

Signs of Restored *Qi*

- Relief of aches and pains
- Reduction in tension and fatigue
- Mental clarity
- Feelings of well-being and peace of mind
- Adequate energy to complete tasks

While massage practitioners use finger pressure and muscle massage to promote healing, acupuncturists use micro-thin needles. These needles are relatively painless, although during a treatment one may experience a needle prick, a feeling of pressure, or other momentary sensations. After the treatment, the intensity of pain usually diminishes or the pattern of pain changes. The healing process will take more time and energy when damage and disability are great. The possibility of increased pain exists for a short period of time when the life force increases the healing process in long-standing or more difficult problems.

Acupressure Massage

Massage, the oldest Asian healing art, originated in Central China. Today in China people receive acupressure treatments in the form of gentle *Anmo* (按摩 sounds like "ahn moe") massage and firm *Tuina* (推拿 sounds like "two+we nah") therapy. The Japanese combine acupressure with massage in a way that relaxes the body while energizing it. This lively therapy is called *Shiatzu*, which translates as 'finger pressure'—*Shi (ZHI* 指) means 'finger,' and *atzu (YA* 壓) means 'pressure.' The acupressure practitioner stimulates reflex points, massages muscles and flexes the frame in order to restore balance and harmony, increase vitality and promote health. Acupressure massage is simple, safe and effective for people with a variety of lifestyles. Anyone can realize the far-reaching benefits of regular acupressure treatments using the methods detailed in this book.

Acupressure can benefit acute and chronic conditions and prevent disease by strengthening the immune system. Acupuncture is especially effective with more painful chronic conditions. The stimulation of reflex points can alert the practitioner to sore spots indicating an imbalance in the person's system. These early warning signs present an opportunity to correct the condition before a more serious complication occurs.

People in all walks of life, especially those who experience tension and stress from work, can benefit from acupressure.

Who Benefits from Acupressure?

- An executive might notice increased mental power
- An athlete may find increased endurance, flexibility and fluidity
- A student may find it easier to concentrate on studies
- Everyone can better deal with challenges and frustrations

Acupressure massage is preventive medicine when used regularly. The stimulation of reflex acupoints alerts the individual to the presence of sore spots. These early warning signs indicate an imbalance in the system. Acupressure helps to maintain health and prevent disease.

Disease-Preventing Benefits of Acupressure

- Restoring balance and harmony
- Increasing the life force
- Strengthening internal organs
- Helping the immune system fight disease

Bacteria, viruses and other seeds of disease are always present. Incorrect living habits lower our resistance, thereby allowing microorganisms to grow and thrive. No external precautions in the form of antiseptics or face masks can prevent illness when our internal environment is ripe for disease.

Acupressure massage is therapeutic, increasing the flow of blood and lymph, which carry off toxins and bathe the tissue in a fresh supply of life-promoting oxygen and vital nutrients. In this way, *Shiatzu, Anmo, Tuina* and other therapies from the Far East encourage natural healing.

Therapeutic Effects of Acupressure

- Eases aches and pains
- Reduces tension and fatigue
- Promotes deep satisfying sleep

Acupressure massage is rejuvenating. Life's tensions can cause us to feel sluggish and older than we are. A treatment leaves you feeling relaxed and energetic—in a word, younger.

Rejuvenating Results of Acupressure

- Improved memory and clarity of thought
- Increased vitality and stamina
- Greater precision and ease of movement

As a technique for promoting health and well-being, acupressure can be an important part of a balanced program of self-development. Massage adds another dimension to communication, bringing people closer together through the power of touch. Asian healing arts remove blocks to the free flow of energy and reinforce the life force. People feel more energetic because degeneration is reversed. Acupressure is something you can do on a regular basis to promote good health.

The Chinese have a saying, "There are three treasures in life: health, wealth and friends. Of these three treasures health is the most important. Without health you cannot enjoy the other two." To prolong life and promote health, *The Yellow Sovereign's Classic* advises, "Never fell your own trunk, nor attack your own roots." The body is a marvelous organism, always striving towards growth and health. However, most of us are constantly hacking away at our life force unknowingly through our choice of lifestyle. Often we take in food and drink that poison rather than nourish us. We fail to heed the signals from our body to relax or to exercise.

Chinese Philosophy

The mythical father of Chinese practical philosophy, Fuxi (伏羲 traditional date -2852), proposed the theory of yinyang as a guide to gaining knowledge, categorizing information and predicting the future. Many Chinese still believe that studying the relationship between patterns of light *(yang)* and shade *(yin)* can be used to predict the future. Can you predict the future? Wouldn't it be nice if the future were predictable? Well, some of it is very predictable. Surfers use tide tables. Monday begins the workweek and Friday ends the week, except for holidays. Holidays change according to the date or the day of the week every year. Calendars help predictability. If we agree to meet next year on Wednesday, September 29, you can predict with some confidence that the meeting will happen a year from now. When a soap opera is on at 11:00 A.M., advertisers count on millions of Americans being in front of the TV at that time. You can take that to the bank—and they do.

This year a springtime rainstorm blew our almond blossoms off the branches to the ground. The beautiful sad scene of blossoms on the ground painted by the rainstorm looked like snowfall. We could not have predicted the rainstorm, but we could predict a shortfall of almonds this autumn.

On Wall Street, commodity and stock traders look at the fundamentals: interest rates, energy prices, labor strikes and storm damage; then they predict whether a stock will move up or down. The storm was very destructive this year, so the price of almonds may go up and someone will put money on the line. They say it's like gambling but traders swear they fare far better than gamblers. Predicting it will be daylight tomorrow at 10:00 A.M. is not telling the future, it's common sense. But daylight tomorrow at 10:00 A.M. is not certain. We could be knocked out of orbit by a cosmic event.

The theory of *yinyang* can help you predict the future when doing massage on people. If you know how to evaluate the situation and treat appropriately, you are more likely to elicit the outcome you desire. Just as I can predict the outcome of a massage, I can predict that in four hours I will be in the next town. I know the way, and I have a car, so unless something catastrophic happens like an accident, or I am pulled over by a cop who thinks I look like the guy featured on "America's Most Wanted," I will arrive in four hours. If, in your mind, no one can predict the future, you might redefine that statement somehow and say, "No, he's just estimating probabilities."

Many of the fathers of Western experimental science once believed if you knew the laws of matter and energy you could predict the future. Early in the 1800s the scientist Marquis de Laplac theorized we live in a completely deterministic universe. He proposed if one knows exactly 'what is,' and the laws governing it, one can accurately predict the future like an expert billiard player. To prove a theory one sets up an experiment and predicts the outcome. Many things are more predictable because of experimental science.

The *I Ching*

The *I Ching (Yijing* 易經 sounds like "E ching" the *Classic of Change)* is a book about *yinyang* relationships. It categorizes social situations and offers sage advice on the appropriate action. The *I Ching* warns people against consulting it to predict the future. Instead, people are advised to consult this classic of divination to receive advice on possible courses of action and the resulting consequences.

Psychologists today listen to and advise clients about how to overcome disorder(s) in their lives, making life more predictable. Diviners, astrologers and psychics past and present, like psychologists, counsel people about the possible consequences resulting from their actions. The *I Ching* reads like a psychologist's notebook with principles of behavior and case histories. Some of the case histories are of the concerns of ancient Shang and Zhou kings.

An ancient legend alleges that in prehistoric times the sage-king philosopher Fuxi developed a classification system to predict the future. He was the leader of a nomadic tribe whose members hunted and trapped. This tribe also made strong cords for nets and fine threads for clothing. With nets they could catch more elusive game and carry things in bags. Fuxi used knotted cords as an accounting system and he invented the written pictograph. Two symbolic diagrams are attributed to him:

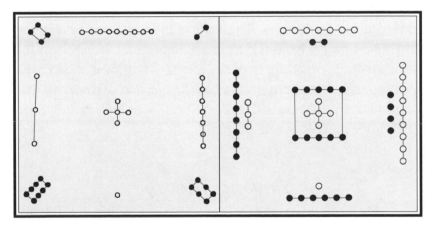

4	9	2
3	5	7
8	1	6

The knotted cord diagrams (above) represent numbers arranged either as a magic square (combinatorial number pattern) or as a cross. Anthropologists do not know when in high antiquity the magic square appears, but the Chinese used the magic square long before any other civilization. The oldest form known is nine numbers arranged in a three by three checkerboard which add up to fifteen in all columns, all rows and main diagonals.

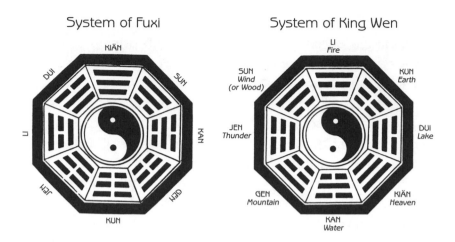

| System of Fuxi | System of King Wen |

The Bagua (sounds like "bah gwah") or Eight Trigrams (above) and the magic square of Fuxi shown previously are remarkable documents. The Bagua is found on the Korean flag. The images for the Bagua are listed clockwise from the twelve o'clock position: heaven, wind (wood), water (stream), mountain, earth, thunder, fire (bright) and lake (marsh). The Bagua commonly classifies directions, seasons, hours, family members, colors and animals.

Yinyang Theory

China's mythical First Sage-king Fuxi established a community in China's great basin of the Yellow River. He contemplated the world around him to make sense of its apparent chaos. He observed that dark night and daylight alternate daily, noted the inhabitants of the world respond to this rhythm. The long cold winter is followed by a hot season. The two extremes of light and dark, and hot and cold, alternate periodically but not identically. Plants become active in the warm season, resting under ground in the cold season. The activities of animals and people harmonize with the daily and yearly cycles. Activity and sleep harmonize with the daily cycle of day and night. In the summer, when it's hot and the days are long, humans tend to be more active, while in the winter, when the days are cold and the nights are long, we tend to pursue mental activities. Exceptions to the rule exist, as some people and animals are active at night. Both extremes are necessary to life. Fuxi saw these extremes as complementary opposites. One limit he called yin, the other yang.

From this understanding, Fuxi developed the unifying principle of *Yinyang*. The Chinese language is ideographic,

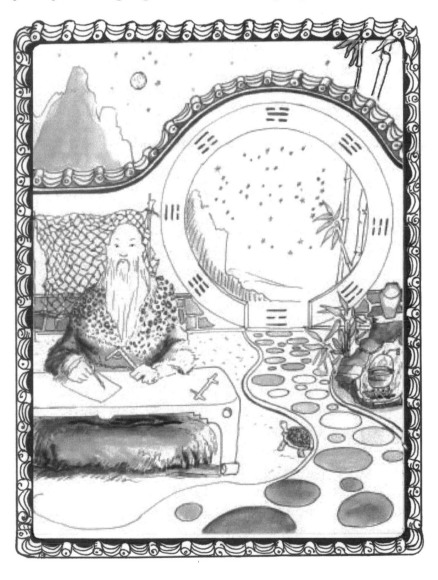

so it is natural for words to be composed of images. The ancient Chinese character for *Yin* (陰) depicts the shady side of a hill; the character for *Yang* (陽) depicts the sunny side. In *The Yellow Sovereign's Classic* the image of *Yin* is water; the image of *Yang* is fire. With this principle, Far Eastern cultures found order in the world around them. Winter does not last forever; the sun will again warm the earth to awaken the life within. Eventually, the warm and light fade, and it is once again winter, the time of rest.

The image of water falling to the earth from the skies as cooling rain, seeking the low places, forming pools and lakes and eventually traveling to the ocean is *Yin*. Pure water can be obtained from the earth by digging a well. The *I Ching* is a source for many Chinese sayings. One of these reads, "You can relocate a city but you cannot relocate a well."

The image of fire rising from the earth to heaven as currents of air visible as smoke or mist is *Yang*. Vapors rise when water evaporates on a sunny day. Fire burns wood from the outside in as it heats the air that rises up. Water is used as an image in many Chinese sayings and teachings such as, "Water drips through rock." Water is so soft, yet it has the power to wear through rock (a good thought for those afflicted with chronic disease).

Other common Chinese sayings are:

"Water floats a ship and sinks a ship."

"With enough fire you can cook anything; with enough money you can do anything." Water and fire can be used to create or destroy depending on how folks use them.

"Distant water cannot stop a near fire."

"Real gold fears no fire."

"No paper can wrap a fire," is being said, I imagine, today in reference to China and the Internet.

"Water and fire do not mix." Interesting how we notice when opposites attract like magnets.

Yinyang Patterns

	Yin (陰)	*Yang* (陽)
The Light	Dark	A Light
A Day	Night	The Day
Season	Winter	Summer
Temperature	Cold	Hot
Direction	North	South
Image	Water	Fire
Altitude	Low	High
Sequence	Before	After
Sound	Quiet	Loud
Realm	Earth	Heaven
Species	Plant	Animal
Being	Body	Mind
Stuff	Matter	Energy
Supply	Deficit	Surplus
Depth	Inside	Outside

All living things, when young and healthy, are supple and soft; when old and diseased, they become rigid and hard. Yinyang describes life as existing between these two poles. Once you understand the idea of yinyang and see how opposites are not only antagonistic but also complementary, don't stop there. To stop there is to see a tree and say, "I have seen a forest." Opposites define each other. The contrast can be used to understand the whole. Opposites are unstable, always changing ... day and night ... winter and summer ... life and death. Life and death are not opposites, they are irreconcilable differences forever intertwined. You can't live with it and you can't live without it. When one sees opposites as complementary, one principle works with the other to perfect the whole.

Historically, Western civilization has seen the same phenomena and called it duality, not unity. Light opposes darkness from this point of view. Water and fire are antagonistic, not complementary. It took Western science by surprise to learn from Albert Einstein that the realm of matter and the realm of energy were not separate and conserved, but could be converted one into the other. The opposites of matter *(Yin)* and energy *(Yang)* are now seen as complementary and comprise the whole of space-time *(Yin-Yang)*.

Yin, imagined as the force of water, is cooling, with a preference for rest, shade and the inside of things, also referred to as *Yinqi* (陰氣). Water controls fire and can extinguish it. *Yang,* imagined as the force of fire, is warming, with a preference for activity, light and the outside of things, also referred to as *Yangqi* (陽氣). Fire controls water and can evaporate it. In the heavens, the fiery sun evaporates the oceans of water, creating weather. Activity and rest change the earth. *Yinqi* and *Yangqi* represent generalized complex conditions in terms of traditional Chinese sciences.

This concept can be extended to the healing arts as well. Fire (energy) and water (matter) come together at conception and separate after death; their interplay sustains life.

Western medical tradition has viewed the mind (energy) and the body (matter) as separate entities. Similarly, the Western symptomatic approach to treatment pre-supposes that the body is a collection of separate parts, each of which can be treated alone. By contrast, Asian medicine, which is based on the *Yinyang* principle of unity, treats the mind and the body as complementary aspects of a whole. The practitioner of Asian medicine focuses on the entire body, rather than a single diseased part. This approach is reflected in the current trend in the United States toward wholistic medicine. An old idea is being born anew.

Yinyang Patterns

Acupressure massage applied without evaluating a person's *yinyang* nature, or without noticing the *yinyang* characteristics of the tissues being worked (massaged, stimulated, etc.), limits the value of the treatment. Various *yinyang* combinations are commonly found. The *yinyang* of the disease factors should be considered in relation to the *yinyang* constitution of the person. Disease can pass through several stages and many causes can occur together, and their signs and symptoms overlap. Tailor each treatment to fit the individual and adjust each treatment depending on the state of health and stage of disease. More complex *yinyang* relationships are a greater challenge to an acupressure therapist. This is how we learn.

People are *yin* or *yang* depending on their sex, disposition, age, activity (work or play), body build and (temporarily) the *yinyang* nature of their disease.

Yinyang of Constitutions

	Yin (陰)	*Yang* (陽)
Sex:	Female	Male
Build:	Frail, fat	Husky, lean
Life style:	Mental	Physical
Disposition:	Introvert	Extrovert
Age:	Very young/very old	18 to 40-60 yrs.
Complexion:	Pale	Reddish
Judgment:	Intuitive	Intellectual
Nerves:	Hypoactive	Hyperactive
Temperament:	Depressed	Irritable
Body while resting:	Curled up	Stretched out
Voice:	Quiet	Loud
Breathing:	Short and weak	Coarse

If you think someone is pure *yin* and you cannot see the *yang* in him or her, you have not seen all there is to see. All people have both *yin* and *yang*. *Yin* and *yang* are polar characteristics. They are the theoretical extremes. Nothing is pure *yin* or pure *yang*: all things are combinations.

The *yinyang* characteristics of a person's constitution and state of health will determine the treatment. *Yang* people need deeper, more vigorous treatments, while yin people need lighter, more gentle treatments. When the disease is *yin*, the treatments should be (*yin*) more gentle; but if the disease is *yang*, work (*yang*) more firmly.

Yinyang of Disease

Modern term:	Eliminative	Degenerative
Characterized by:	discharge	weakness
Modern medical term:	acute	chronic
Duration:	short term	long term
Energy Quality:	*Excess*-True	*Deficient*-False

The presence of chronic disease indicates the body is weak and not functioning properly. Weakness *(yin)* can lead to a new disease, causing the body to muster more energy *(yang)* to eliminate the new disease. When our immune system is weak, we get sick more often, depleting even more energy. Sometimes we may not completely recover, which leads to more serious diseases.

Degeneration takes place subtly—we become accustomed to it. Our bodies lose a little flexibility, circulation decreases and waking up takes more time. Recovery takes longer; we feel new aches and pains. We tell ourselves we are getting older and the problems are minor. We just can't do as much; we have to 'take it easy.' We forget the little bit of lost 'aliveness.' We settle for our new state of health, though we can't do what we could do before, whereas an Oriental medical doctor would diagnose a *deficiency* of energy.

There are two main types of disease, eliminative *(yang)* and degenerative *(yin)*. Both have the same source, which is an imbalance of energy within the body. When the life force is strong and active *(yang)*, the body eliminates *excess*. Eliminative disease is a process by which the body normalizes itself by eliminating toxins and their accompanying microorganisms. The symptoms are discharges and fever recognized as the symptoms of colds, infections and flu.

Degenerative disease occurs when the life force is weak *(yin)* because the eliminative *(yang)* process has been inhibited. When a body cannot discharge or neutralize toxins, the organs and tissues function only partially or shut down and cease to function, resulting in cancer, heart disease, and a host of other chronic and serious disorders. Many times, other organs take over or supplement the functions of the diseased organs. This, of course, puts an added load on the helping organs, and if the balance is not restored, these organs will also degenerate.

The body can heal itself and has an immune system for defense. To a healthy body, light massage and heavy pressure are both acceptable during a session. This is not true during illness. To help the body heal itself, a treatment can be gentle or vigorous and use light or heavy pressure depending upon the disease producing factors. The length or treatment time and frequency will vary.

The ancient Chinese discovered that degenerative or chronic diseases are caused by a *deficiency (XU* 虛 sounds like "shoe") of energy. While acute disease results in an *excess (SHI* 實 sounds like "sure") of energy. The two terms combined indicate the quality of health. The term *XUSHI* (虛實 sounds like "shoe sure") is defined as 'the actual situation.' For our purposes it translates as 'quality.' The English word quality usually categorizes and quantifies the nature of something. If you consider the quantity of something as part of its quality, then the word quality is a true translation of the compound term *XUSHI*.

Individually the words *SHI* and *XU* describe both quality (true/false, real/facade, honest/deceitful) and quantity (excess/deficient, solid/empty). The full range of meanings is even greater. *SHI* is defined as (1) solid; (2) true, real, honest; (3) fact; (4) fruit; (5) eliminate, discharge, acute, new or short duration. *XU* is defined as (1) void; (2) empty; (3) in vain; (4) timid; (5) false, deceptive; (6) humble; (7) weakness, poor health; (8) theory; (9) virtual, facade; (10) degenerate, chronic, old or long duration.

Quality Pattern

	SHI (實)	XU (虛)
Degree of disease:	excess	deficiency
Health is:	true	false
Modern term:	eliminative	degenerative
Characterized by:	discharge	weakness
Modern medical term:	acute	chronic
Duration:	short term	long term

When you have true *(SHI)* health your diseases are of the *excess (SHI)* type and you will acutely discharge toxins, pain and pathogens. Then your immune system truly becomes educated and you build solid *(SHI)* health. When you have false *(XU)* health your diseases are of the *deficiency (XU)* type and your weak health continues to degenerate *(XU)* chronically. High quality health means you enjoy being active and have greater quantities of energy for rapid healing. Low quality health means your energy is low and you will probably be depressed and suffer poor quality healing.

With *excess* pain you can predict that as long as the body's healing energy is not suppressed, the pain will be eliminated. In the case of *deficiency* pain, the body does not have the resources to eliminate pain. Even if it's the mildest of pain, you can predict that more pain awaits you in the future.

The body can easily eliminate *excess* even if the pain is intense. The body cannot get rid of *deficiency* without help. The *deficiency* needs to be supplemented. *Deficiency* pain does not mean the pain is deficient it means the body is *deficient* in energy to eliminate the pain. *Excess* does not

68

mean the pain is excessive, it means the body's energies are strong and the pain will be eliminated (discharged).

To summarize, an *excess* pain does not mean a severe pain and a *deficiency* pain does not mean a mild pain. *Excess* pain means 'easy to get rid of.' *Deficiency* pain means 'hard to get rid of.'

Change Pain into Energy

The idea of the 'life force' (called *Qi* by the Chinese) includes the process of changing disease into health. *Qi* energy is the key to understanding the body's self-healing power. If the ancient Chinese are correct and pain is injured *Qi*, that changes everything, including the way Westerners evaluate and treat pain. If pain is our life force working to heal injuries and infections, then suppressing pain will have tragic consequences, such as chronic debilitating pain and disease. Now is the time for all good people to come to the aid of their bodies. Now is the time for a reevaluation of how we treat pain by learning more about energy.

The Chinese written character for *Qi* 氣 includes two images—that of steam 气 above grain 米. Steaming grain, the image of cooking, represents the most common life-transforming activity people perform. The idea behind the word *Qi* represents the 'life force' as a process rather than an entity. Observing the stages of a process differs from examining things and their parts. When examining parts in ever-increasing detail, a machine-like theory of life evolves. The Western metaphor views the body as a machine. In contrast, the Chinese metaphor views the body as an energy system. The study of process reveals functional activity and the interaction of parts within a whole. Activity uses energy over a period of time. Through careful study of the transforming nature of *Qi* energy, the practice of Oriental medicine was developed. Chinese physicians diagnose the patterns produced in the struggle between health and disease.

To understand the Asian concept of health and disease, *Qi* energy must be seen as a process rather than a part used in healing. To think of energy only as something that flows from the universe to you—through the body from practitioner to patient, or from patient to practitioner—limits the creative process of the activity to that of a technical repairman. The theory of *Qi* in Oriental medicine proposes that studying the stages of disease and the stages of healing will lead to the knowledge of the process, therefore accelerating healing and establishing glowing health.

The ancient Far Eastern sages taught that all disease comes from problems with the flow of *Qi* and *blood*. *Stagnant Qi* and *congealed blood* result from disease, causing pain. To help the body rid itself of disease and pain, find the painful spots, then press until you feel the *Qi* energy moving. When the therapist moves the *Qi*, accelerating the healing process, the patient experiences *Qi* sensations.

The term *Move Qi (DAOQI* 導氣 sounds like "dow chee") combines the Chinese character *DAO* (sounds like "dow") meaning to lead, to guide, to teach, to persuade, with the character for *Qi*. *DAOQI* refers to the process of inducing and directing *Qi* by stimulating acupressure points in various ways to transfer energy along the channels. The process results in *Deqi* meaning *Got Qi*.

The term *Got Qi (Deqi* 得氣 sounds like "duh chee") combines the Chinese character *DE* (sounds like "duh") meaning to get, to effect, with the character for *Qi*. *Deqi* is a word used to express the experience of *Qi*. During acupressure the feeling of *Qi* is experienced as a radiating, glowing, flowing sensation. *Deqi* is obtained during acupuncture when the patient feels a sensation perceived as sore, aching, electric, tingling, numbing, heavy or swollen. The acupuncturist also feels the *Qi* energy as it 'grabs' the needle. One of the basic concepts of acupuncture is that *Deqi* is necessary for effective treatments.

The term *Stagnant Qi (QIZHI* 氣滯 sounds like "chee jee") describes the first stage of disease wherein *Qi* energy pools at an acupoint, along a *meridian* or anywhere in the body. When *Qi* energy is stuck, the *blood* will *congeal* unless energy is moved through the area. The image of the Chinese character for *congeal* is silt at the bottom of a river. *Congealed Blood (YUXUE* 瘀血 sounds like "you shoe+way") accompanies or follows *Stagnant Qi. Stagnant Qi* is often experienced as a sharp pain. *Congealed Blood* is felt as a dull ache.

The Yellow Sovereign's Classic, Volume I, "Simple Questions," chapter 5, titled "The Grand Theory of the Reciprocal Nature of Yinyang," states **"Pain is injured *Qi*"** or "*QI SHANG TONG* (氣傷痛 sounds like "chee shang tong")." The body tries to restore the flow of energy when the life force stagnates. Injuries to the life force hurt and it takes energy to remove the blockage. Therefore, one has less energy for other activities.

The body shows signs of stress while healing. If it had a voice it would say, "I need your help." Slow down or stop other activities. Use the time to help speed healing. There are three ways to create a healing environment within your body: (1) increase the circulation of *Blood* and *Qi* energy through acupressure massage and acupuncture, (2) eat healing foods and (3) breathe pure air.

Pain announces the presence of serious *Qi* stagnation in the body which signals information about the intensity and location of stagnation. There are two ways to stop pain. One is to slow or stop the healing response with pain-relieving drugs and the other is to accelerate healing. Benjamin Franklin once wrote, "Men take more pains to mask than mend. Bad gains are truly losses." Pain warns you to slow down while healing is taking place. Masking pain robs you of your life energy. The problem is not pain. The problem is how to best assist healing. When *Qi* energy heals, pain warns and directs the healing response. Nurture *Qi* energy to speed healing. Pain can be used to evaluate a disease. It is not the disease, nor is pain just an annoyance that accompanies disease. Pain is the body trying to heal itself while sending signals that can be used to speed healing.

Do not mask pain; you will know healing is complete when there is no pain. In the hands of a skilled practitioner, pain can be useful to resolve the disease process at its roots.

When disease blossoms, pain appears.

The Chinese word for pain is pronounced *TONG;* the image of the character is one of 'disease 疒 blossoming 甬.' The theory of 'Roots and Branches' in *The Yellow Sovereign's Classic* suggests that disease, like a weed in a garden, has roots and branches. The root is the cause and the symptoms form the branches. The disease blossoms into pain and will persist if you remove just the symptoms—leaving the root. By using drugs to remove the flowering pain without observing its message, more pain is sure to follow. For example, a gardener learns to perpetuate flower production by picking the blossoms before they become fruit, then the plant quickly produces more blossoms.

Plants are identified primarily by examining the parts—branches, leaves and blossoms—that are above the ground. (The symptoms and the pattern of painful spots reveal the cause of the disease.) When the root of a pain is eliminated, the pain and symptoms disappear. If pain returns, one must continue to search for the root, healing the diseased tissue at its source.

Blocked energy stagnates, forming a reserve that people experience as pain. When we unblock this stagnant energy and allow it to flow, people may feel energy sensations. Disrupted energy pathways can be empty *(Deficiency)* or full *(Excess);* either can create problems. Block a river by constructing a dam and the excess water behind the dam stagnates, while a deficiency of water below the dam starves the land. The stagnant water behind the dam kills trees, bushes and other plants. Fish dependent on the flowing river and animal life on the banks become endangered. Fish and plants adapted to living in stagnant water will replace the life forms that flourished in moving water. Downstream from the dam, the plants and animals dependent on the rise and fall of the river will disappear.

Now we will consider a practical use for these concepts. Make it a habit to evaluate pain before, during and after a session. Evaluate a person's pain to determine the type and intensity. First determine if the pain warns of *excess* or *deficiency*. *Excess* is usually an acute health problem or an acute episode in a chronic disease. *Deficiency* is usually chronic disease or the period of recovery following an acute illness or injury. *Sedate* the *excess,* using vigorous acupressure like *Tuina,* or *tonify* the *deficiency* using gentle massage movements like *Anmo.* Ask about the intensity of the pain. (Refer to the **Pain Intensity Scale** on page 84.)

The Root of Pain

A guiding principle is: *external* (表) pain indicates the use of the *meridians* that pass through the painful area. *Internal* (裏) pain indicates the use of acupoints on the limbs and back that affect the internal organ responsible. A healthy diet and the proper herbs strengthen the internal organs.

The *external* body includes the skin, limbs, head and *meridians*. The *internal* body includes the internal organs and glands. Disease can send roots throughout the body. The prime directive is: eliminate the root—eliminate the disease. However, to relieve discomfort, first treat the symptom, then treat the root. *External* disease usually results from infection or injury, trauma, environmental conditions or changes in the weather. *Internal* disorders usually result from imbalance caused by extremes of life style, poor diet, or inappropriate emotional expression.

If health problems do not heal completely, a deeper cause of disease is indicated and the internal organs must be treated. Nutrition and life-style counseling beyond the scope of this book should be sought.

Our *external* body is directly affected by environmental conditions including: changes in the weather, exposure to the elements, overwork and trauma. The *external* body can take great abuse and recover easily if the internal organs are healthy. *External* disease is usually mild with a short recovery time. *External* problems can injure the *internal* organs when the defenses are weak. This is referred to as the **penetration** of disease. An example of an *external* disease is a cold or flu. The symptoms include fever, headache, nasal congestion and avoidance (dislike) of cold or wind.

Diseases of the *internal* organs have different patterns than those of the *external* body. When the body's balance between *yin* and *yang* is upset, the *internal* organs are directly affected. The food we eat and the emotions we express upset our *yinyang* balance. *Internal* disorders can cause *external* body problems that are difficult to treat. They usually are more severe and last much longer. Recovery from *internal* disorders occurs slowly and may not be complete. When the body's resistance to disease is low, it indicates *internal* weakness.

A pain with a deep root is treated differently than a pain with a root in the *external* body. The Chinese theory of roots and branches suggests that pain and disease are like weeds in a garden. To eliminate a weed, destroy its root. Masking a pain, even with acupressure, will allow a disease to continue, resulting in more pain. Just as relieving pain without consideration of the root results in more pain, a gardener knows picking flowers encourages the plant to produce more flowers. To eliminate pain treat the root.

When gathering information, consider the evidence of an injury or infection. Feel with your eyes and look with your fingers. Let your heart guide your fingers; the way to treat reveals itself. Look for the root of a pain, then choose the points based on its location. Select the acupoints by the depth of the pain. The root of a pain is either located in the *external* body or the *internal* organs. The following is a simple guide to find the root of pain.

External (表) Pain

Signs: Pain mostly in extremities: head, arms and legs
           Sometimes back pain
           Most back pain is due to an underlying weakness
           Injury and invasion tend to happen at the weak
           places
           Recent onset or flare-up of old problem
Therapy: Locate the *meridian* (see *Meridian ID and Location*
           chart on page 94) nearest the pain or injury
           Select acupoints (page 200) along the *meridian*
           near and distant

Internal (裏) Pain

Signs: Pain mostly in trunk: abdomen, chest and back
           Sometimes joint pain
Therapy: Locate the diseased organ (see **Acupressure
           Therapy** on page 205) (if you don't know, find a
           doctor who can locate the root of disease)
           Select associated acupoints on arms and legs
           Rub and press the back near the diseased organ

Some time ago a runner came to see me. She said she injured her knee while running and the way she described it made sense to me. After six treatments on her knee, the pain was gone. She came back six months later and said the pain was back. I realized I had missed the root of the pain. I observed the painful point was where the Gallbladder (Gb) *meridian* crossed the knee. This time I tested every point on the Gb *meridian* up to her hip but found nothing remarkable. Pressing points down to the foot, the acupoints were not tender until I pressed Gb.42. She reacted with a start and I asked her if she knew that point was sore. She said no. I treated that point only and the knee pain disappeared. I saw her years later and the pain had never returned. The root of the knee pain was in the foot. It is interesting to note that books on acupressure or acupuncture treatment do not mention Gb.42 for knee pain.

The Quality of Pain

A guiding principle is: weekly gentle treatments for chronic diseases and daily aggressive treatments for recent injuries and infections.

Distressing pain is an urgent message to stop and do something now. Mild pain is a reminder something is wrong—look for the root. Pain is not the disease. Pain is your body healing the disease. It needs help. Improve the quality of your energy and the quality of your pain will improve. The quality of pain is often directly proportional to the quantity of pain and often indirectly proportional to the intensity of pain. Pain begets energy; they must be the same. An ancient Chinese proverb states, "Dragon begets dragon; phoenix begets phoenix."

Pain, in the mind of an Oriental physician, is injured *Qi* energy. When the pain is *excess* the body is actively healing the problem and, if given the opportunity, the body will heal completely and the pain will not return. If the healing process is interrupted, the pain will become chronic.

Pain often includes *yin* and *yang* aspects. *Internal deficiency* makes it more difficult to heal *external* pain. If your symptom pattern indicates an *internal* disease and you are unaware of a diseased organ, see a doctor who can locate the root of disease. Have a medical doctor diagnose which organ is diseased, unless you have already been diagnosed. Once you know which organ is diseased, locate the organ in the body. Feel for sore spots in the muscles and joints near that organ.

'Acute' and 'chronic' are terms describing pain in the West. An acute pain is a recent sharp pain with rapid onset, whereas a chronic pain is a longstanding pain with slow progression, often thought to have no treatable cause. These terms are similar to two terms used by Oriental physicians. Though they are not identical, they can help you evaluate the quality of pain quickly. The two qualities of pain are *excess* (similar to acute) and *deficiency* (similar to chronic). *Excess (SHI 實 sounds like "sure")* and *Deficiency (XU 虛 sounds like "shoe")* guide in the application of *tonification* or *sedation*. (See the following section **Treating Pain** and the section **Shiatzu Movements** for further guidance on *tonification* and *sedation.*)

Chronic pain occurs when the energy of the body is frustrated with the healing process. *Excess* (acute) pain results from a new injury or invasion. *Deficiency* (chronic) pain results when the healing process has fatigued. An *excess* pain occurs during a *deficiency* disease when the healing process renews its attempt to heal the chronic disease. *Deficiency* (chronic) pain, though mild, is more difficult to eliminate. *Excess* (acute) pain, though severe, is easier to eliminate.

In Chinese medicine an *excess* pain can blossom from a *deficiency* disease; these pains can be relieved with *sedation*. However, to eliminate *deficiency* pains for good, the cause of the *deficiency* must be supplemented with herbs and/or diet. The advice of an Oriental physician may be sought.

The best way to assist in healing new and chronic pain:

Excess (SHI 實) Pain

Indications: A new problem or a flare up of a preexisting one
Hurts worse when first worked; relief comes slowly, but improves daily
Pain 'hurts bad,' does not improve easily

The way it feels after a traumatic injury, like a bruise

Observations: Tissue looks swollen

Skin looks red

Feels warmer than surrounding area

There may be a discharge

Therapy: Daily treatments using *Sedation* techniques:

First use strong pressure on acupoints distant from the area

Then press gently (if at all) on the painful spots

Increase vigorous massage in the area around the problem

Always avoid pressing hard directly on the most painful places

Deficiency (XU 虚) Pain

Indications: An old pain and soreness

Feels good to be worked. Some say 'it hurts good'

Always gets relief, but does not improve over time

The way a muscle feels after doing a new exercise routine or starting a vigorous activity after some time off

Similar to the soreness you feel the day after skiing or hiking for the first time that year

Observations: Skin discolorations and small colored spots on skin around problem

Feels like a pattern of stiff and soft flesh

There is weakness and poor circulation

Therapy: Weekly treatments using *Tonification* techniques:

Massage around the sore area to work out the pain

Acupressure on hard stiff spots; massage on soft tissue

Disease results when the drive to be whole encounters imbalance, injury or infection. If there is no *internal* organ *deficiency*, disease cannot invade the *external* body. Many serious diseases start with flu-like symptoms. A cold or flu leads to an *excess* of energy as the body resists because of the initial *deficiency*. When the body's defenses are lowered because of a *deficiency*, one is more likely to get a cold or flu or more serious disease. With lowered resistance, it leads to an increased risk of degenerative disease. When your defenses are up, viral and bacterial diseases can be avoided.

Twist your ankle and it responds with excess fluid and fire. It feels hot and swollen. It will go away unless the body's healing process is reduced. *Deficiency* pains start as *excess* pains. First there is an *excess*, the body tries to heal and if it cannot, you are left with a *deficiency*. The healing process can be restimulated with a mild reinjury such as acupressure or acupuncture.

After an injury, the body's healing process maximizes within one day and begins to fatigue after four days. Healing continues for a few more weeks. A stimulating little reinjury will renew the healing for another four days. A serious reinjury will cause more damage. This can happen when the pain is masked with drugs, herbs or even acupressure. Once the healing process has completely fatigued, you are left with a *deficiency* problem.

I have had patients who have had several serious injuries in the past with very little pain left in their bodies. They are the type that did not like pain pills (which mask pain); they used heat and rubbing to soothe their pain and cautiously became more active. They did not baby their pain and they did not ignore their pain; taking these actions would reinjure the painful place in little ways that restimulates the healing process. Acupressure and acupuncture are small injuries that provoke a healing response. They are informed ways to reinjure and accelerate healing.

The Color of Pain

A guiding principle is: acupressure when *hot* (熱); massage when *cold* (寒).

Appearance can help diagnose the true cause of pain and disease. When working on a body, notice skin coloration of various parts overall or very small spots. New scars are often very red and old scars are often paler than the surrounding skin—they do not have pigment. The face is often a different color than the rest of the body. The same is true of the palms and the soles of the feet; they often change color more quickly. The face can change color more quickly than the body. It becomes red with embarrassment and anger. It becomes pale with fear or melancholia. Facial complexion can tell you something about the present state of emotions.

The Chinese discovered the body displays signs to help determine the best treatment method. Observe the color of the skin around the area of pain, but also look at the face and hands. Color reveals the most likely therapeutic movements needed to relieve the pain. It also reveals much about the state of health. Does the area around the pain or the whole person look hot or cold? Look at the appearance to determine the best therapeutic movements: acupressure or massage.

Heat applied to the body increases circulation and promotes relaxation. Heat relaxes *Qi*, but too much heat injures *Qi* and the body becomes exhausted. Cold firms the body but too much cold injures the body and the body swells. Today some people believe in a recent idea that cold reduces swelling. But consider this: cold reduces the circulation of blood and lymph, depriving the injured tissue of nutrients from the blood and the removal of waste by the lymph. All living tissue needs a fresh supply of food and regular elimination of waste. The use of ice and cold reduces circulation and therefore postpones healing and results in prolonged swelling. An acupressure massage increases circulation, which accelerates healing and therefore reduces swelling after an injury better than ice or cold. The use of ice and cold is like the use of pain and anti-inflammatory pills, which give relief today, but you must pay the price in the future.

You can place your hands on the top and bottom of another's hands or feet (like a 'hand sandwich') and feel a difference in temperature. If the palms are hotter than the backs of the hands, it is an indication of a *yin deficiency*. If the palms are cooler than the backs of the hands, it is an indication of a *yang deficiency*.

Hot and cold signs can also indicate a *deficiency* of the body's *yin* or *yang* energies. *Deficiency* of *yin* water shows signs of *heat*. *Deficiency* of *yang fire* shows signs of *cold*. Determining *excess* and *deficiency* are necessary in interpreting *hot* and *cold* signs. A body may look *hot* or *cold* everywhere or areas may look hot or cold. Treat all or part accordingly.

Hot (熱) Pain

Signs: Pain relieved by cold (use cooling therapy rather than cold or ice)
Red skin
Dry, rough skin

Therapy: Press and pinch

Cold (寒) Pain

Signs: Pain relieved by heat (use warming treatments, a little heat is okay)
Pale skin
Moist, oily, soft tissue

Therapy: Rub and stroke

Note: Some believe that cold reduces swelling and pain but, as with pain pills, it only postpones healing, which results in more prolonged swelling. Increased circulation achieved with acupressure and massage will reduce swelling after an injury more effectively than ice or cold packs.

In the West, we are attracted to fiery women. To be attractive, women paint their cheeks red and apply dark outlines to their eyes. These customs create the appearance of disease. One of the signs of disease in Chinese medicine is a malar flush. It is a sign of a serious chronic *yin deficiency*. Indications of a malar flush on the cheeks are small red veins marking the skin creating the appearance of rosy cheeks. Dark circles around the eyes also indicate a serious chronic *yin deficiency*. Makeup masks our true feelings and may conceal signs of disease. Appearance may be deceptive. A malar flush, at first glance, may look like a spontaneous blush, but one is chronic and the other is acute.

Heat applied to the body increases circulation and promotes relaxation. If you burn yourself it feels hot, the skin reddens, the blood flows faster to carry away the heat to cool the tissue and a blister may form: *fire* produces *water (yang* changes to *yin)*. If the blister breaks, it will weep. Burning yourself with fire or hot things irritates tissue, which causes the body to react.

People look very red as a result of sunstroke caused by staying in the hot sun too long. This is called *excess* (true) heat caused by an *external excess*. Some people look hot all the time. For example, alcoholics often look sunburned, this is a *deficiency* (false) *heat* caused by an *internal yin deficiency (water* fails to control *fire)*.

Cold applied to the body reduces circulation and slows metabolism; the body becomes stiff. The most exposed parts of the body such as the ears, fingers and toes become cold first. The body will recover from cold without damage as long as it does not freeze or the exposure last too long. If it freezes, the tissue becomes brittle, with no circulation, no metabolism. If this condition is warmed and treated promptly, one will recover. However, tissue damage will be extensive when frozen for a prolonged period of time. After the body part is unfrozen it becomes red, hot and painful. The *cold* becomes *hot (yin* changes into *yang)*.

People look very pale and stiff as a result of exposure to the cold. This is called *excess* (true) *cold* caused by an *external cold excess*. Some people look pale all the time. For example, diabetics often look cold, this is a *deficiency* (false) *cold* caused by an *internal yang deficiency (fire* fails to control *water)*.

The healthy body tries to maintain balance so that when one goes out in the cold, more heat is generated. When hot, the body sweats to cool off. When too cold, the body shivers to generate heat. Exposure to the cold can cause a chill that may turn into a fever. This is called *yin* turning into *yang*. Exposure to the heat will bring on a fever that may later turn into chills. This is called *yang* extreme becoming *yin*.

Many people come for treatments within hours after an injury. One woman limped into my office for her regular *Shiatzu* treatment. She said, "I don't know if I should be here or the emergency room." She went on to tell of tripping over the cat and twisting her ankle, which resulted in swelling and pain. When I examined her foot, the anklebones were barely visible. I assured her that she had made the correct decision. After I used the techniques of rapid healing given earlier in the book, she walked away without a limp. The next week she reported being aware of the pain from the injury healing only a few times afterwards.

Treating Pain

The Horse Whisperer by Nicholas Evans is a novel about a cowboy philosopher who tames wild horses. It begins with a terrible accident that maims a young girl and her horse. The horse, driven mad by pain, must be helped or destroyed. The legendary Tom Booker, who trains horses with voice and touch, offers hope. Tom disagrees with horse tamers who inflict pain to train horses. His philosophy is to use a horse's natural response to pain to heal the animal.

Horses are sensitive animals whose first response is to flee pain but then turn to face it, like a teething baby who does not avoid pain but bites on it (page 255). Injured horses often get worse before they get better (page 266). Tom's success came from the idea that pain is both hope and healing. He said, "... where there's pain, there's still feeling and where there's feeling, there's hope" (page 289).

Stimulating an acupoint causes both a local and a distant effect. After pressure is applied for a short time, a local change takes place. The energy increases at the acupoint where pressure is applied. The distant effect is minimal until more pressure is applied or more time passes. Generally, it takes pressing for one to three breaths before a distant effect is achieved.

The amount of time and pressure applied affects the healing response. More time and/or greater pressure changes the healing response from strengthening called *tonification (BU* 補 sounds like "boo"), to calming called *sedation (XIE* 瀉 sounds like "she+ah"), to the extreme of numbing analgesia *(MA* 麻 sounds like "mah"). Nourish and protect the life force by learning to tonify, sedate and stop pain.

To Tonify: Increase the energy at an acupoint or location
               Use less pressure and more time
               Watch for increased circulation: skin feels warmer,
               looks redder, while the muscles feel more relaxed
To Sedate: Decrease the energy at a distant acupoint
               Use more pressure for less time
               Skin feels cooler: there is reduced redness and
               even greater muscle relaxation
Analgesia: Use more time and more pressure
               Pain is stopped or reduced

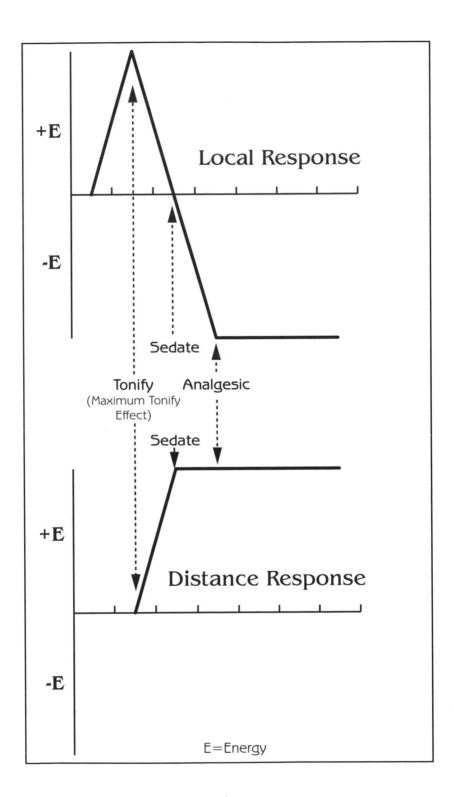

85

The following scale can be used to evaluate pain before and after a treatment as well as days later to determine the effectiveness of the treatment.

Pain Intensity Scale

Intensity (Quality): Description

Mild (Annoying):	Not noticed when person is active but is evident when a person is relaxed. Usually tender, dull pain
Uncomfortable (Tiring):	Person will tire more quickly, lose energy. Usually a sharp, sore pain
Distressing (Miserable):	Less tolerable than the previous two. Affects view of life and is noticeable by expression on face. Usually piercing pain
Horrible (Intense):	Person is motivated to do something (anything) about it
Excruciating (Blinding):	Too painful to move. Also described as splitting or crushing

People may feel energy sensations when the painful acupoints release their reserves of *Qi* energy. These *Qi* sensations *(Deqi)* are usually mild. Strong sensations may be experienced if a person has robust *internal* energy that has been severely blocked. The following scale of sensations will guide you in evaluating the intensity of the energy flow.

Deqi Energy Scale

Intensity: Sensations

Mild:	Warm, tingling, fullness, expansive
Moderate:	Glowing, itching, numbing, flowing
Strong:	Burning, prickling, heavy, electric

If a person feels more than one point radiate to the same area, that area should be examined for injured energy.

Shiatzu Movements

There are four basic movements in acupressure massage:

- Rub (*AN* 按 sounds like "ahn")
- Press (*MO* 摩 sounds like "moe")
- Stroke (*TUI* 推 sounds like "two+we")
- Pinch (*NA* 拿 sounds like "nah")

The movements are easy to learn and produce an effect far beyond the effort required to perform them. In *Shiatzu*, a little effort goes a long way.

There is no one **right** way to perform the basic *Shiatzu* movements. Begin by practicing each movement as it is explained here. As you develop your individual style and gain experience, modify your technique to suit the situation.

Giving a *Shiatzu* massage should benefit you as well as your partner who receives it. You know you are performing the movements properly if:

- You feel comfortable, rather than awkward
- You feel energized, rather than drained
- The motions seem effortless, rather than arduous

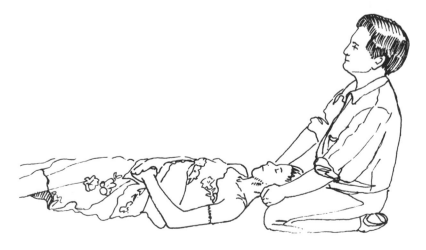

To **rub** *(AN)*, move the skin in quick circular motions using the pads of the fingers or heel of the hand. Rubbing is used to stimulate the surface and middle tissue layers.

For finger circles, your hand should be slightly cupped, with the fingers straight and firmly held together. Rotate your hand and arm from the elbow in a counter-clockwise direction if you are right-handed or clockwise if you are left-handed. Use just enough pressure so that your fingers do not slide on the skin. Push the skin around in big circles over the muscles for the length of one breath, then move to an adjacent area and repeat. Your free hand should rest gently on the body.

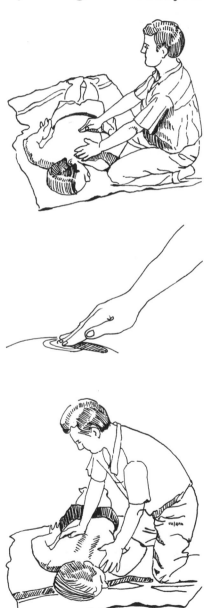

To use the heel of your hand, place both hands on your partner's body with the heel of the working hand in the middle of the area to be stimulated. Keep your fingers relaxed using your arm and shoulder to push the heel in a circle—again, counter-clockwise if you are right-handed or clockwise if you are left-handed.

To **press** *(MO)*, apply continuous pressure to an acupoint without moving. The fingers, thumb, or heel of the hand can be used to press an acupoint.

Finger pressure uses the pads or tips of the fingers to apply light pressure to stimulate an acupoint near the surface. To apply pressure to a small area, use one finger or place one finger on top of the other. To apply pressure to a larger area, place the fingers side by side. The fingers are most often used to press points on the face, neck, abdomen, sternum and ribs.

Thumb pressure uses the pad, or first joint of the thumb to apply heavy pressure to a relatively small area. To press with the thumb, your body should be balanced and centered. Your arm should be straight but not locked. When

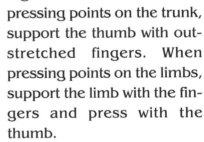

pressing points on the trunk, support the thumb with outstretched fingers. When pressing points on the limbs, support the limb with the fingers and press with the thumb.

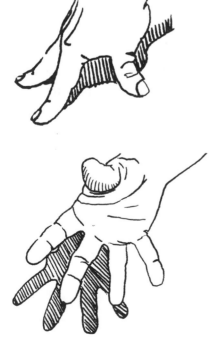

To **stroke** *(TUI)*, press and slide the skin forward and backward along the length of the muscle. Use this movement repeatedly to massage an acupoint or to break up ropiness in a muscle on the back, buttocks, legs, or shoulders.

To apply light pressure, use the finger pads. For deep pressure, use the thumbs. Place your thumbs on the acupoint or area to be stimulated, stretch out your fingers to support the thumbs.

Pull the skin toward your fingers, alternating thumbs with each pull.

To **pinch** *(NA)*, grasp a muscle with your hand in the form of a pincher (four fingers together opposed to the thumb), squeeze and then release. When possible, exhale as you squeeze the muscle, inhaling as you release (see section on Centering page 198). This movement can be done slowly and firmly (holding the muscle for one to three breaths, releasing slowly) or rapidly and vigorously (pinching and releasing once or twice per second).

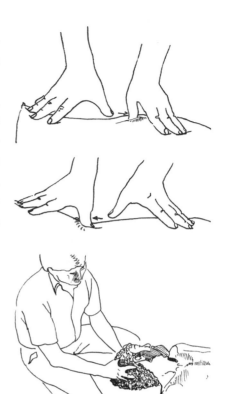

By shifting your body weight, you can vary the amount of pressure you are applying as you perform the various movements. A **light** *Shiatzu* is used to evaluate an area and to treat sensitive points. To give a light

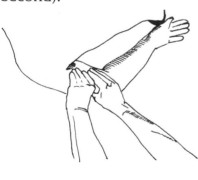

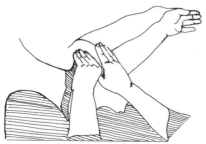

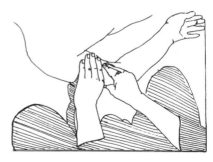

Shiatzu, work on the surface, using large circles, fast rhythm and light pressure. A **moderate** *Shiatzu* covers a smaller area, uses smaller circles, a slower rhythm and more pressure. A **deep** *Shiatzu* probes the gray area between pleasure and pain. It resembles the sensation of working out the soreness in an aching muscle. For a deep *Shiatzu,* press acupoints firmly, holding or stroking slowly. A Chinese proverb entreats, "Slow work; quality work."

Although your fingers are your main tools in *Shiatzu,* they are only channels for the *Qi* energy flowing between you and your partner. You should give *Shiatzu* with your entire body, focusing weight and consciousness at your fingertips.

Acupoint Basics

Acupoints are pressure-sensitive areas along the fourteen primary channels of energy that run through the body. The acupoint location describes a place on the skin—not the acupoint itself, which is found between the skin and bone. Its exact location is known because of its sensitivity to touch. Pressure on some acupoints will produce a local sensation, while on others, a sensation may be experienced at a distance.

The fourteen energy channels are functional groupings of acupoints. Twelve of the channels are *meridian (JING 經* sounds like "jeeng") pairs duplicated on each side of the body. Two are channels *(MAI* or *MO 脈* sounds like "my") which run along the midlines of the body, both front and back. Ten *meridians* are named after internal organs, such as the spleen and liver. Two *meridians,* namely the *Circulation-Sex* (Cs) and the *Triple Heater* (Th), are associated with the functions of blood circulation and water distribution in the body respectively. Two *meridians,* the *Vessel of Conception* (Vc) and the *Governing Vessel* (Gv), coordinate the energy flows in all of the *meridians.*

The acupoints receive their names from the *meridians* they are on, however they may have only a slight, if any, influence over the organ or function in their name. The relationship between the energy channels and the organs or functions for which they are named is beyond the scope of this book. Remember, just because an acupoint is named after an organ, i.e., *Bladder* 10, the acupoint is not necessarily associated with that organ.

Each of the twenty-eight acupoints in this book are identified in five ways:

(1) by the traditional Chinese characters, (2) by a transliteration of the traditional Chinese pronunciation in *PINYIN*, (3) by a translation of the Chinese name in **bold italic**, (4) by a nickname in Small Caps and (5) by an abbreviated acupoint identifier using two letters, a dot and a number, i.e., Bl.10.

The abbreviated acupoint identifier is most useful for identifying and locating acupoints. This system (used by Western acupuncturists and some acupressure practitioners) is similar to an early method of abbreviation developed by the French, who were the first Westerners to take a serious look at acupuncture. They found it necessary to simplify the traditional Chinese point names, because of the difficulty in translating and understanding the archaic names. Today, with increased knowledge of ancient Chinese, acupoint names are thought to describe the location or traditional function of an acupoint. In some cases, the original meaning of the characters has been lost.

People often assume because an acupoint is named after an organ, that the acupoint has something to do with the organ; in fact, it is seldom true. The Chinese do not and never have used the organ serial numbers to identify the points (examples of the Chinese names are given in the section on acupoints). Therefore, the Gallbladder *meridian* is not the gallbladder. The Kidney *meridian* is not the kidney. They are distinct and separate. It is better to think of them as having nothing to do with each other. The numbering system to identify acupoints with an organ and a number has caused confusion for many people learning acupressure.

The abbreviated acupoint identifier used in this book begins with a capital letter, followed by a lower case letter and a number. The letters refer to the name of the energy channel along which the acupoint is located. The number refers to the location of the acupoint along that *meridian*. For example, Co.4 refers to the fourth acupoint along the *Colon meridian*, which runs from the tips of the index fingers, up the arms, along the top of the shoulders and up to the sides of the nose.

The abbreviated acupoint identification system is not used to describe the function of the various acupoints. For the ten *meridians* named after the internal organs, only some of the acupoints along the portion of the channel on the arms and legs have a direct influence over those organs. For example, soreness in Co.4 may indicate constipation. Pressing that acupoint has an effect on the function of elimination. However, the acupoints on these *meridians* will also affect other organs and functions. Most acupoints do not directly influence the organ or system implied in the name. For example, Bl.17 is the seventeenth acupoint on the *Bladder meridian*, but it is not directly associated with the urinary bladder.

To avoid confusion, look upon the acupoint identification system as a list of street addresses that can help you find your destination but does not provide a description of the occupant.

Next to the Chinese names, which are of historical interest, are nicknames that I have used as a teaching tool in my classes. Some of the nicknames are from Chinese sources; some have been suggested by my students and colleagues; many I have made up myself.

Meridian ID and Location

ID	Meridian	Location of Pathway
Lg	Lung	*Yinqi* flows from the chest to the hand
Co	Colon (Large Intestine)	*Yangqi* flows from the hand to the face
St	Stomach	*Yangqi* flows from the face over breast and belly to the foot
Sp	Spleen-Pancreas	*Yinqi* flows from the foot to the chest
Ht	Heart	*Yinqi* flows from the chest to the hand
Si	Small Intestine	*Yangqi* flows from the hand to the head
Bl	Bladder	*Yangqi* flows from the face, down the back to the feet
Ki	Kidney	*Yinqi* flows from the foot to the chest
Cs	Circulation-Sex	*Yinqi* flows from the chest to the hand
Th	Triple Heater	*Yangqi* flows from the hand to the face
Gb	Gallbladder	*Yangqi* flows from face down the side of the trunk to the foot
Lv	Liver	*Yinqi* flows from the foot to the chest
Vc	Vessel of Conception	Reservoir of *Yinqi* on the front midline of body
Gv	Governing Vessel	Reservoir of *Yanqi* on the head and back midline of body
S-	Special Acupoint	A non-*meridian* acupoint

To the ancient Far Eastern healing masters, blemishes like pimples and warts are a sign of blocked energy nearby. Both a history of diseases and a current disorder can be read at acupoints by observing freckles and pimples or other skin marks. When body marks are found it is thought to be a good sign that the body's energy system is correcting itself. Body marks such as freckles and moles are thought to be a sign that the body has healed itself in the past. Pimples are a sign that the body is eliminating and healing itself in the present.

Four Acupoints
for a Healthy Self

"It's your lantern, don't poke holes in the paper."
"There's no place like happiness or sorrow—find them in yourself."
—Chinese proverbs

Pain goes when energy flows. The following four acupoints are essential energy points. They are easy to locate and will relieve pain throughout the body. They also benefit *Qi* and *Blood*. They will balance *Yinqi* and *Yangqi*, as well as, strengthen digestion, improve elimination, increase circulation and strengthen immunity for everyone who uses them regularly.

"The doctor of the future will give no medicine but will interest his patients in the care of the human frame and in the cause and prevention of disease."
—Thomas Alva Edison

氣海

QIHAI

Energy Ocean

Vc.6

The Chinese name for Vc.6 (Vessel of Conception 6) is transliterated as *QIHAI* (sounds like "chee high") in most modern English texts. In older texts, if it is mentioned at all, *QIHAI* is probably written as *Ch'i Hai*. Either way, it means **Energy Ocean**. Two Chinese characters represent *QIHAI*. Previously the character for *Qi* was described as an image of vapor above grain revealing the nature of *Qi* energy. The *Ocean* character belongs to the *Water* group, modified by the concept 'every.' Every drop of water arose from the ocean and seeks to return to the ocean. This notion flows from the image of *HAI (Ocean)*.

Chinese written language reveals images rich in symbolic meaning. Chinese writing from earliest times used pictographic (line drawings) and ideographic (pictographs combined to represent abstract ideas) images called characters. We use phonographic images called letters, which are combined to represent things and abstract ideas. The Chinese characters are drawn with one or more brush strokes, representing a basic idea. The meaning of most characters can be understood by considering the placement of small icon-like figures one on top of the other, side by side, or in multi-icon groupings. Complex characters have a 'Group Icon' figure called a 'radical' (the root of the idea) modified by an 'Object Icon' figure referred to as a 'phonetic' or a 'specifier.' The radical (Group Icon) and the specifier (Object Icon) together make up complex characters.

Characters in a Chinese dictionary are grouped by the radical (Group Icon). Radicals represent categories with images such as: human, earth, water, wind, fire, mountain, wood, rain, valley, river, ocean, shell, fish, sun, crops, plants, field, moon, flower, flesh and disease. Chinese dictionaries group characters into over two hundred categories. The number of characters found in a category varies from a few to several hundred. There are over one hundred large categories of characters.

The character *HAI* (海 *Ocean)* is a complex character that includes three images: *Water*, *Person* and *Breasts* (mother). It combines *Water* (氵) as a radical next to 'every' as a specifier. The 'every' character is a common specifier used in constructing Chinese characters. The 'every' image has a *Person* (𠂉) icon above and a *Mother* (母) icon beneath. It can be said every person has a mother—the one thing that each human has in common with all other humans is a navel. Just as every person came from a mother, every drop of water in rivers, ponds and lakes came from and will return to the ocean. Likewise, in people, the source of all energy is a vast reservoir in our abdomen referred to as *QIHAI*, ***Energy Ocean***. The Chinese character *HAI* also means vast, extensive and accumulative (as the ocean).

Vc.6, ***Energy Ocean,*** is the most famous acupoint for energy. The Chinese gave this acupoint nicknames like 'the Light of Life' and 'Elixir Field' *(DANTIAN* 丹田 sounds like "dahn tee+ ahn"). These terms refer to a field, an ocean, or a domain of the life force. Stimulating this acupoint releases origi-

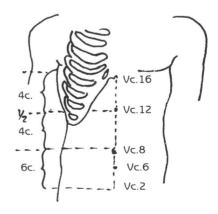

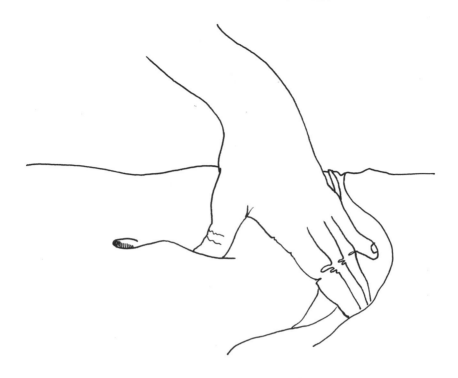

nal undifferentiated energy. This energy is used for healing but can also be used for other activities essential to life such as respiration, circulation and digestion as well as non-essential activities like playing in sports or playing around.

Energy Ocean, Vc.6, located on the front midline of the body, is found two fingers width below the navel. The acupoint is the sixth on the *Vessel of Conception meridian*, a *yin energy* channel designated a *Blood Ocean meridian*. *Blood* is *yin* and *energy* is *yang*. It is said the *yin blood* nourishes *energy* and the *yang energy* commands *blood*. The *Conception Vessel (Yin)* located on the front of the body is paired with the *Governing Vessel (Yang)* on the back of the body. The *Governing Vessel* is designated as an *Energy Ocean meridian*. A stronger *Yinqi* will support a stronger *Yangqi*. Fitness experts point out that strong abdominal muscles support a strong back. Therefore *Energy Ocean* is located on the *Blood Ocean* meridian. *Blood* nourishes *En-*

ergy and *Energy* commands *Blood*. *Yin* supports *Yang* and *Yang* directs *Yin*.

The *Vessel of Conception* has twenty-four acupoints on the front midline and no acupoints on the arms and legs. The central *meridian* acts as a reservoir, channeling *Yinqi* through crossing acupoints directly to all the *yin* channels. At their ends, the *yin* energy channels change into *yang* energy channels. A general principle from *The Yellow Sovereign's Classic* states after *yin* reaches its maximum it changes into y*ang*; after *yang* reaches its maximum it changes into *yin*.

Abnormal *Qi* is either *excessive* or *deficient*. The sensation goes **upward** from this acupoint indicating *excess Yangqi*, or a *yin deficiency (false heat)*. This upward flowing *Deqi* energy can go to the *liver* or *heart* to indicate healing energy is needed there. Energy flowing **downward** from the point indicates an *excess Yinqi,* or a *yang deficiency* (false cold). *Yang deficiency* can be inherited from parents or acquired by burning the candle at both ends. As a person improves with treatments, the energy may consistently flow in **both** directions spreading a great distance indicating normal *Qi*. It may be difficult to press Vc.6 and achieve a *Qi* sensation on yourself.

Energy Ocean (Vc.6) is buried deep within the abdomen. Under the muscles and connective tissue are the small intestines. Under this acupoint toward the feet is found the urinary bladder and the uterus (in women). To the sides are the ascending and descending colon. Toward the head are the transverse colon and the stomach.

CAUTION: **Never apply pressure directly to a pulsing object in the abdomen.** The abdominal aorta feels like a pulsing cord—stopping the flow of blood through it will cause great damage. The artery is easily felt and easily avoided. **If you suspect weak or frail arteries, or have an existing aneurism, check with your doctor before receiving a massage.** There is nothing to fear when receiving massage from an experienced professional, but be sure to tell them of your condition.

Prepare the abdomen by rubbing *(AN)* the skin over the muscles, then focus your massage below the navel. Warm up the area, pressing *(MO)* deeper with a slower rhythm and smaller circles; you will soon be pressing Vc.6, the **Energy Ocean** point. Locate **Energy Ocean**, Vc.6, two fingers below the navel. Press with your thumb, but not too hard. Move slowly, allowing the body to receive your thumb. When you feel a slight resistance, hold for a few breaths. How does it feel? You may feel a throbbing above or to the side. The abdominal aorta is near, but as long as you do not feel a strong pulsing directly below, you can press deeper. However, before you press deeper, allow the release of tension, then gently move your thumb back and forth so you can feel that it is actually in between those deep muscles called the psoas. At the deepest level, if the body will let you in, you may press against the bones of the spine or the sacrum. After you have held the acupoint at the deep level for one to three breaths, come out and gently rub the area.

Press into the **gray area** between pleasure and pain so the receiver can feel energy moving. Typically, the first sensation felt is pressure in the abdomen a small distance away from the **Energy Ocean** point. Adjust the force with which you apply pressure. If the point becomes more painful, press lighter; if the point becomes less painful, press with greater force. When you press, press in gently. You can rub deep in the abdomen as long as pain is not distressing. Pain indicates blocked energy. Blocked energy comes from emotional tension, long-term energy depletion, chronic disease or other violations of the laws of life.

If you work just right, you may be able to release energy that your partner feels moving and working in the body. Energy sensations may be distant from where you are pressing. A common sensation is of pressure or a throbbing radiating feeling or simply tingling. Some people feel it go **up** indicating *excess yang* or *yin deficiency*. This is quite common because our culture encourages hard work and discourages rest. When people burn the candle at both ends, the fire depletes the water, which brings a condition known as *yin deficiency* or *YINXU*. Other people feel energy sensations moving **down** indicating *excess yin* or *yang deficiency*. Also, where energy sensations go can indicate energy needs for a particular organ. When energy is balanced and flowing without blocks, it may be sensed circulating upward and downward equally, indicating good health.

Key concepts to remember about Vc.6:
- CAUTION: Never press on a pulsing artery in the abdomen
- Location: Two fingers width below the navel (Vc.8), along the front midline
- Deqi: Everywhere (especially stomach, genitals, low back)
- Use: Promote longevity. Release vital energy for strength and healing. Fill energy reserves. Regulate use of *yinyang* energy. (Also stops bleeding, regulates menses, benefits the spine, strengthens digestion, aids elimination, warms hands and feet, regulates water metabolism)
- Pain: All types (especially abdominal, bladder, emotional, menstrual)
- Condition: Menstrual problems, bladder infection, depression, fatigue, constipation, infertility, bloating

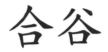

HEGU

Joining Valley

Great Eliminator Co.4

Co.4 (Colon 4) is the most well-known acupoint and often misused by the non-professional. Read carefully how to press this point to feel its power. Many people know that this acupoint can relieve pain, especially headaches. They also often know the Chinese name, *HEGU* (sounds like "ha goo") or *Hoku*, even though they have no knowledge of other acupoints. The first character *HE* means 'to join, to unite, meeting, adjoining.' The second character *GU* means 'a mountain pass or a mountain valley.' Translation of *Hegu*, **Joining Valley,** reveals the secret of how to press this acupoint for the strongest energy response.

HEGU also evokes associations to the great river valley of China. Chinese ancient history records how people cultivated and civilized areas along the Yellow River *(Huanghe* 黄河 sounds like "who+ahng ha"). This great river basin and vast flood plain provided fertile ground for producing food. The Yellow River floods also brought great destruction at times. Another danger to the farmers living in the valley came from nomadic herdsmen. The northern mountains proved to be a natural obstacle against invading bandits, who used the mountain passes to access the riches of China along the Yellow River. The reason the Chinese built the Great Wall was to 'head them off at the pass.' Defending mountain passes helped eliminate the threat of invading tribes. *HEGU* stimulates the immune system to defend against invading microorganisms.

The nickname, GREAT ELIMINATOR, fits this acupoint well because it aids elimination from the bowels, eliminates congestion in the head and excels at eliminating pain. This point boosts the *Yang* immune system's ability to eliminate colds and flu. It becomes sensitive when the immune system battles invading microorganisms even before the first symptoms appear. Co.4 is also used to reduce fever, relieve pain, clear the skin, stop spasms, diminish tension, clear a stuffy nose and decrease toothache. A nickname in the West is 'The Dentist's' point because it can stop tooth pain and moisten the throat and tongue.

Another name for the point is TIGER'S MOUTH. Hold the hand out in front of the body with the thumb at the bottom. Open and close the space between the thumb and hand so the thumb acts like a tiger's lower jaw; the acupoint is deep in the tiger's mouth.

The name *Joining Valley* advises how to position the hand to get the most powerful energy response by joining the thumb to the hand, making a mound with a valley. The best way to locate Co.4 on yourself is to place your palms on your stomach. As you close the space between your receiving hand and thumb, notice the mound of flesh on the back of the hand and the crease in the mound. Locate Co.4 at the end of the crease, near the middle of the mound. Keep the thumb against the hand as you press *(MO)*. Place your pressing thumb on the end of the crease, massaging the mound of muscle against the bone of the hand. Feel the muscle roll around under your thumb. Massage the muscle against the

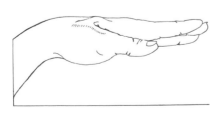

hand bone to feel for sore spots. What does the muscle feel like? Does it feel hard? Does it feel soft? Does it feel like stringy strands? Can you feel lumps in the muscle?

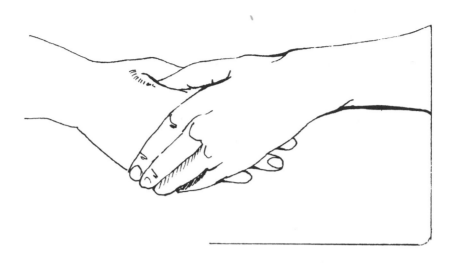

IMPORTANT: **press this spot into the bone of the hand**, slowly sliding the tip of your pressing thumb along the bone. Slide along the hand bone toward the index finger for a short distance and then toward the wrist. Slide back and forth **until the most sensitive spot** can be felt. Press firmly on this spot. This point may be **very** sensitive. Sensitivity can make it easy to find, but you will have to work slowly to achieve an energy sensation. When the point is not sensitive you will have to press harder to find it, but it is easier to get the energy sensation.

Moving Qi can be easy at this acupoint if you take your time. Stop and hold the acupoint. Does energy move outward from the point? It may travel to another spot in the hand or the arm of the hand being pressed may feel a sensation move upward. The *Qi* sensation may be felt around the elbow or even the shoulder or head. When you increase pressure, the *Qi* sensations become stronger. If you increase the time the point is pressed, more varied sensations may be felt.

The *Colon meridian* starts at the tip of the index finger. It passes along the side of the index finger closest to the thumb. Midway along the hand bone (second metacarpal), the path dips into a depression in the large muscle (dorsal interosseus) that forms the web of the thumb; this deep location near the middle of the hand bone is where Co.4 can be found. The *meridian* then passes between the tendons and muscles on the thumb side of the wrist and forearm on its way to the elbow.

The *Colon meridian* crosses the elbow at Co.11, the shoulder at Co.15, the neck at Co.18 and ends on the face, next to the nose, at Co.20. The *Colon meridian* includes points numbered Co.1 through Co.20, as well as Gv.14 and St.37. The *meridian* also passes into the trunk connecting with the lungs, colon and stomach. Areas along the path can benefit from stimulating Co.4.

This *meridian* supplies *Yangqi* energy to the head, neck, shoulder, arms, colon and lungs. Co.4 is the *Source Point* (*YUAN* 原 sounds like "you+ahn") on the *Colon meridian*. Acupoints designated as *source points* derive energy from *meridians* with which they are coupled through *Connecting Channels* (*LUOMAI* 絡脈 sounds like "Lew+oh Moe"). *Yinqi* flows into the *connecting channel* and *Yangqi* flows out. The *yang Colon meridian* receives *Yangqi* energy from the *yin Lung meridian* that obtains *Yinqi* energy from the lungs. The *Lung meridian* receives fresh energy from the lungs through the acupoint *Central Treasure* (see Lg.1 on page 123), where the deep circulation of energy comes to the surface. After flowing down the arm toward the wrist, the *Lung meridian* crosses a *connecting channel* at Lg.7 where the energy passes into the next *yang meridian*, the *Colon*, at its *source point*, Co.4. This point can stop pain along the path of the *Lung meridian*. It benefits most problems of the elbow, shoulder, neck and head.

Co.4 is an important healing acupoint associated with many body functions. Stimulate it to restore *yang* energy, to improve digestion, elimination and immunity. This point is also one of the easiest to use to create a *Qi* sensation that moves up the arm. Most people will be able to generate this sensation on themselves and others by remembering the secret given in the name ***Joining Valley***.

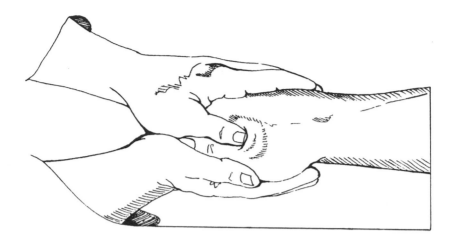

A simple way to locate this acupoint on a partner is to grasp your partner's left hand with your left hand, using your right thumb to press Co.4. Hold your partner's thumb against the hand, look for the crease in the mound and press gently into the crease. Stroke *(TUI)* back and forth along the hand bone to zero in on the acupoint. Remember some people are quite tender here.

Key concepts to remember about Co.4:

- Location: on the hand in the middle of the triangular web between the thumb and index finger
- To find: first massage the web with your fingers, checking for tenderness. Then, hold the thumb against the side of the hand. Notice the crease in the mound. Press at the end of the crease into the mound against the hand bone of the index finger.
- Deqi: up the arm to the elbow, shoulder and head and/or toward the fingers
- Use: Promote longevity. Detect difficulties with and improve *Yang* functions, including sensory organs, immunity and skin
- Pain: all types (especially in the upper body i.e., headache and toothache)
- Condition: constipation, diarrhea, rash, fever, common cold, sinus problems

三陰交

SANYINJIAO

Three Yin Crossing

GREAT YIN Sp.6

The Chinese name for Sp.6 (Spleen-Pancreas 6) is *SAN-YINJIAO* (sounds like "sahn yeen jee+ow"), which can be translated as *Three Yin Crossing*. The nickname is GREAT *YIN*, which reminds me that this acupoint benefits *Yinqi* and all the *yin* organs in the body. This acupoint especially helps women *(Yin)* during menstruation (blood is *yin*) because it relieves cramping and bloating.

Since the 1960s, two of my interests have been backpacking and *Shiatzu* massage. Acupressure has many uses while backpacking. While hiking in the Southern California mountains on a beautiful spring morning, I came upon a young woman who was sitting by the side of the trail with her head in her hands. I stopped to ask what the matter was and whether I could help. Without looking at me, she responded, "I have severe pain from menstrual cramps. I took some aspirin, but it hasn't helped. Do you have some pain relievers?"

I replied, "No, I don't need them. I've studied acupressure. It can be used to relieve most of the symptoms of menstruation. I've used it before. It doesn't always work, but it doesn't take long to try."

I explained how Sp.6 is pressed to relieve the symptoms, and that it usually works within ten minutes. That seemed reasonable to her, so I proceeded. Within a few minutes, she said she was beginning to feel better. After about ten minutes of pressing, she got up, announcing she was pain-free.

109

I explained, "The pain may return, but you can press the point yourself." We talked for a while as she put on her back-pack. We walked the same trail, sharing some of our thoughts and feelings. Before long we parted and my day continued beautifully.

Later, while visiting my mother, I told her about my new interest in acupressure, explaining how helpful it could be. I related the experience of helping the hiker and I demonstrated by locating the acupoint on her leg just above the ankle. She laughed and said, "Oh my, I haven't had to worry about that for years." Months later, I was surprised and pleased when I received a letter from my mom thanking me for showing her the acupoint. She related how her granddaughter complained of abdominal cramps while staying with her during vacation. This was the first time she had experienced menstrual cramping. Grandma shared her experience of the problems unique to females. Not only could she empathize with her granddaughter, but she could also help with the pain by pressing Sp.6.

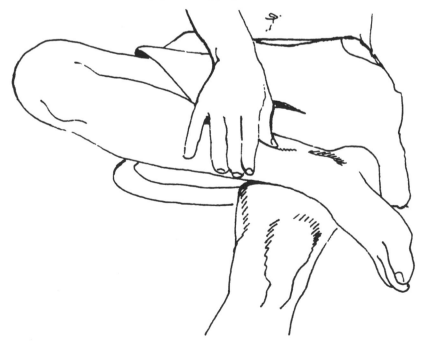

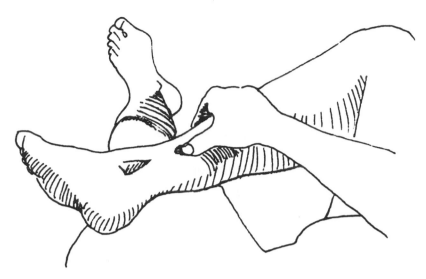

Sp.6 is known as ***Three Yin Crossing.*** I call it simply the GREAT YIN point. When it is sore, there is something wrong with the *yin* energy. Review the various *yin* functions to determine the problem (see **Yinyang Patterns** on page 64).

The Chinese name for this acupoint is another with multiple meanings. The three *yin meridians* that cross here, the Kidney, Liver and Spleen-Pancreas, are thought to be especially important for proper sexual function and for the health of the genitals. The 'three' can also remind you of three broad areas of influence: *Qi, blood* and the reproductive functions.

The character *yin*, in the Chinese name, has many associations. The three *yin meridians* that connect at this acupoint influence all the *yin* in the body: the *yin meridians*, the *yin* organs and the *Yinqi*. The Chinese character *yin* has the image of the shady side of a hill, depicting the idea that the genitals are located in the 'shade' of the human body.

The character for *JIAO* is the image of a person with legs crossed. *JIAO* means crossing, communicating, an intersection, to intertwine. It is an ancient connotation, 'to have intercourse.'

Sp.6 is an acupoint that is tender on women more often than men. Pressure on this acupoint benefits all menstrual

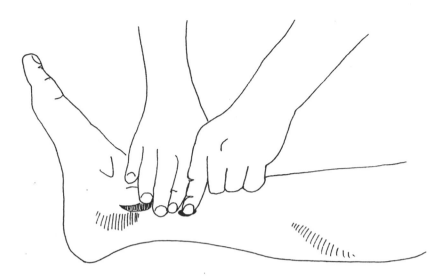

difficulties, urinary dysfunction, hypertension due to *yin de-ficiency*, premature ejaculation, swollen testicles, prolapsed abdominal organs and pain, especially in the low back and knees.

It's easy to locate Sp.6 on your calf. Cross your legs while sitting in a chair by placing your left ankle over your right knee. Massage the muscle behind and above the ankle using muscle pinching *(NA)* and thumb stroking *(TUI)*. Check for tenderness. Find the bottom tip of the inner anklebone (the medial malleolus). With the right hand, measure four fingers above that tip, covering the bony ankle with two of the four fingers. Locate and press *(MO)* into a depression between the muscle and the shinbone.

Look for your partner's Sp.6, which is located a hand's width above the tip of the inner anklebone. Use your partner's hand size to measure this distance. Press into the muscle behind the shinbone on the calf. Press gently at first, because Sp.6 can be very painful on some people. When a woman is menstruating, this acupoint may become tender; in this case, it is then the best acupoint to be pressed. Sp.6 benefits the *yin* and St.36 benefits the *yang*. For balancing energy, press Sp.6 and St.36 (see next acupoint) together.

Key concepts to remember about Sp.6:

- Location: Inside the calf, four fingers above the tip of the ankle-bone
- To find: Rub gently in the muscle behind the shinbone
- Deqi: Up the leg to the knee, thigh and abdomen and/or to-ward the foot
- Use: Promote longevity. Detect difficulties with, and improve *Yin* functions including reproduction and metabolism
- Pain: All types (especially in the lower body i.e., leg and ab-dominal area)
- Condition: Menstrual problems, diarrhea, insomnia, bladder in-fection

足三里

ZUSANLI

Leg Three Mile

GI POINT St.36

The Chinese name for St.36 (Stomach 36) is *ZUSANLI*, which translates as **Leg Three Mile**. This powerfully beneficial acupoint builds strength and endurance. Since ancient times, this acupoint has been used to benefit the legs during long walks; it is the main point to strengthen the digestive system (gastro-intestinal), hence its nickname, GI POINT. There's a pun here, of course; an **army** marches on its **stomach**. The point benefits people with problems associated with standing or walking. When people went for long walks, they would sit down and press this acupoint to relieve tired legs. In Japan, runners, or people with weak legs, use this acupoint regularly to strengthen their legs. St.36 is called the longevity acupoint. It is thought that strengthening digestive energy will prolong life.

The Chinese name for this acupoint has many poetic interpretations. The Chinese character for *ZU* means 'leg,' *SAN* means 'three' and *LI* means a 'Chinese mile' or a 'small farm village.' The image has fields (田) above and earth (土) below. It originally represented the way ancient farm villages looked, with fields laid out in a checkerboard pattern. Later, the character meaning expanded to represent a measure of distance, equal to the length of a standard field.

Farmers cultivate the earth to provide food and herbs— both are essential to keep people healthy. Food and herbs become *Qi* and *blood* that fortify the *internal* organs and

114

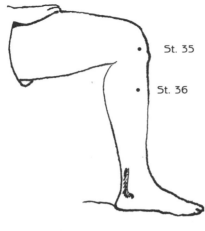

external frame. Since digestion plays a central role in life's activities, St.36 is classified as a *Sea of Nutrition* point. It warns of digestive problems, and benefits the gastro-intestinal tract.

The character *SAN* (three) in the name indicates three areas of influence: the gastrointestinal tract, *Qi* and *blood*. This is an essential energy acupoint. The 'three' in the name also reminds us of its location, three body inches below the knee.

It's easy to find this point while you are sitting down. Notice that when the leg is bent ninety degrees, the knee looks like a cow's nose, with two dents that resemble nostrils. Find the locator acupoint, St.35, in the dent toward the outside of the bottom of the kneecap. To measure three body inches on your leg, use the width of the four fingers on your hand. Measure four fingers down the leg and one finger to the side of the shinbone. The muscles to the outside of the shinbone

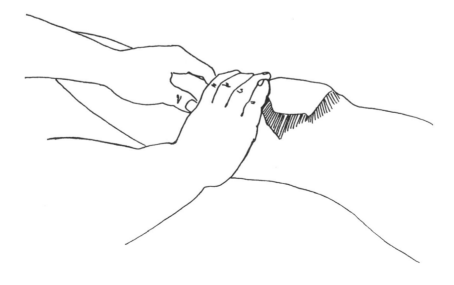

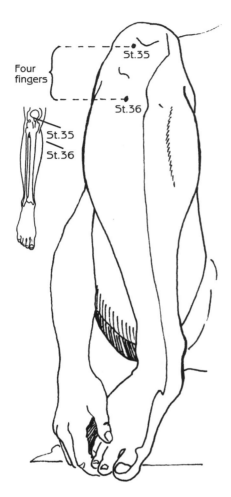

feel tight and, when stroked lengthwise, a separation in the sinews can be felt, revealing a small hole.

Find St.36 on a partner lying face up as follows: use the width of your partner's four fingers to determine three body inches. Sit beside your partner's knee facing the lower leg. Massage around the kneecap. Notice it floats around when it's touched. Make certain it's in the natural resting position when using the kneecap to locate this acupoint. Now find the bottom of the kneecap, feeling where the tendon attaches. Avoid the mistake of measuring from the bottom of the puffy skin below the kneecap; feel for the bony bottom of the kneecap itself. Measure three body inches using the width of your partner's four fingers. While stroking the sinews, one finger to the outside of the shinbone, feel for a small hole in the muscle. Place your thumb over the hole and press.

St.36, *ZUSANLI* shares its name with Co.10 (see the next acupoint), *SHOUSANLI*, **Arm Three Mile,** which has a similar location on the arm and provides similar benefits.

Key concepts to remember about St.36:

- Location: Four fingers below the dent at the side of the knee-cap, in a separation in the muscles outside the shin, one finger outward from the forward edge of the shinbone
- To find: Sit with legs bent 90 degrees, find dent at the side of the kneecap, place four fingers down the outside of the shin, press deeply in the muscles next to the shinbone
- Deqi: Down the leg to the foot and/or up to the knee and thigh
- Use: Promote longevity. Strengthen legs. Detect problems with and improve gastrointestinal functions
- Pain: All types (especially leg and abdominal pain)
- Condition: Anemia, hypertension, high blood pressure, tired legs, allergy, fatigue

Eight More
to Heal Thyself

"If you want dinner, do not insult the cook."
"Do not tear down the east wall to repair the west."
"Adapt the remedy to the disease."
   —Chinese proverbs

The following eight acupoints strengthen immunity to disease and relieve symptoms of colds, flu, headaches, sinus congestion, eyestrain, insomnia and hypertension.

Remember:
Pain goes when energy flows.
Energy increases with relaxation.
First rub, then press, then rub again.
Find the spot then press, hold and release.
Under pressure, energy maximizes within stillness.

手三里

SHOUSANLI

Arm Three Mile

GREAT DEFENDER Co.10

Co.10 (Colon 10) is named **Arm Three Mile** and nicknamed GREAT DEFENDER. The Chinese name suggests that this acupoint is used to strengthen the body as is ZUSANLI (St.36). Like St.36, Co.10 is located three body inches from a bony prominence near the elbow (lateral epicondyle of the humerus). The GREAT DEFENDER (Co.10) is a good acupoint for increasing the body's defensive energy. The immune system will let you know when it is fighting disease because this acupoint becomes sore. It is an amazing early warning system. The day before the onset of symptoms, this point announces, by means of increased tenderness, that the immune system has detected an invader. If you do not take it easy and do not take supplements to boost your immune system, you will likely suffer from a cold or flu.

Co.10 is four fingers from the bony bump outside the elbow toward the thumb. To find this point on yourself, place your left hand on the right side of your navel, while lightly grasping the forearm with the right hand. With your right thumb, stroke *(TUI)* the thick muscles on top of the forearm, near the elbow. If you rub *(AN)* along the line from the elbow toward the thumb, you will feel muscles separate into two groups, then you can feel the bone under the thick muscles. You will find a spot that is more tender than other spots along the bone between the two groups of muscles. Rub this

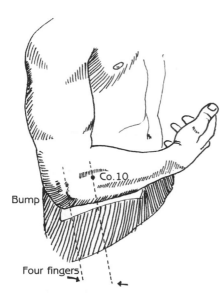

Bump

Co.10

Four fingers

point on yourself every day so that when its sensitivity changes you will know your immune system is active.

To locate on a partner lying face up, place their hand on their abdomen and follow the directions above. You can also leave their arm by their side but the hand must be palm upward. To locate on a partner lying face down, lift the arm by the elbow and place the hand above the head, with the arm bent. With your partner's hand held so that the thumb is up, feel for a separation on top of the forearm in the thick muscles near the elbow. NOTE: Some people have a line parallel to the elbow crease where this acupoint is located. Remember to hold the hand so the thumb is on top.

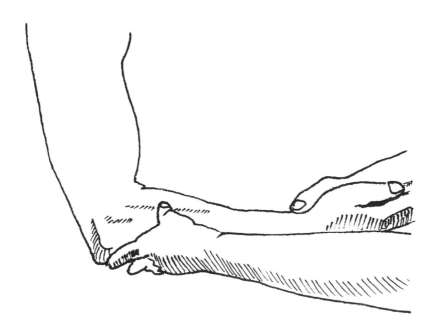

Whether you are finding this point on yourself or a partner, the bones of the arm must not be crossed or the point will be hidden under a large muscle. Notice if you hold your arm in front of you palm up, the bones of the arm (radius and ulna) are uncrossed. You can feel the difference when you turn your palm down; the bones cross. In all the above positions, the bones of the forearm (radius and ulna) are uncrossed. This places the spot on the bone below the muscle separations. Now when the muscles separate into two groups, you can stroke the bone directly under your fingers to find the spot. If the bones are crossed, the most tender spot on the bone will not be easy to find.

Measure four fingers toward the thumb from the bony bump near the elbow, feeling for a small knot above the bone. If that is the most tender spot, the immune system is active. Remember the hand and arm must be in the correct position to locate this point. The acupoint will be lined up directly beneath the separation in the muscle groups, so you can easily press Co.10.

Key concepts to remember about Co.10:
- Location: In a separation between the forearm muscles, four fingers width from the bony bump near the elbow, toward the thumb
- To find: Feel for a small knot next to the bone where the muscles separate
- Deqi: Toward the hand and/or up the arm
- Use: Improve resistance to disease. Strengthen the arms
- Pain: Head, neck, low back (especially pain and stiffness in the arm)
- Condition: Stomach complaints, diarrhea, hypertension

中府

ZHONGFU

Central Storehouse

Lung Lg.1

The nickname for Lg.1 (Lung 1) is simply Lung, but the *Lung* of Asian medicine is anything but simple. The *Lung* is associated with many aspects of health, including a specific time of day, between 3:00 a.m. and 5:00 a.m. The *Lungs* are associated with the season of fall, the flavor of spice and the emotion of grief. The *Lungs* are stressed most during fall. The *Lungs* can be benefitted or harmed by spicy-flavored foods and herbs. When we are sad, breathing becomes labored—we may sigh or sob. Intense or prolonged grieving can damage the *Lungs*. Western scientists have pointed out that during the grieving process we become prone to catching colds and flu; Oriental medicine agrees. Ancient Chinese scientists made dozens of associations with the *Lungs*: color (white), sense (smell), tissue (skin and hair), direction (west), etc. Early in my career, even though memorizing them seemed endless and useless, I discovered the benefits of learning the associations.

One day a man and a woman came to my door asking to talk about religion. I had some time, so I invited them in. I had recently left my job in electronics and was learning about self-employment. I was also studying the application of Far Eastern therapy by working with my massage clients. After welcoming them inside, we had a discussion about God and people. In the late sixties and seventies, my interest in massage and acupuncture, which sounded like 'voodoo' to most Christians, posed problems while attending most churches. I warned them that I was a *Shiatzu* practitioner and talked about healing the body with acupressure energy. They said they didn't mind. The woman mentioned she had a bad shoulder.

I explained the theory of healing using the *meridian* system, which uses energy to heal the body. She agreed to a sample of *Shiatzu* massage. While massaging her shoulder around Lg.1, I noticed a mass about the size of a walnut. As I massaged the lump, I considered what the acupoint **Central Storehouse** (Lg.1) meant in light of my studies. The fact that the lump was painful was a good sign. Energy had solidified at that acupoint. This meant that the acupoint was a potential treasure house of energy. I thought to myself, "What questions should I ask her?" Lg.1 is the alarm point for the lung. The most likely meaning of a lump at the acupoint, **Central Storehouse**, would be respiratory problems. The acupoint is also where newly created energy passes to the surface *meridian* system. This could mean many things downstream from the blocked acupoint. I decided to go with a logical, though less likely, association. The *Five Element Theory* associates the *lungs* with the emotion of grief.

"Have you lost anyone close to you?" I asked.

"Why yes," she said, acting a little shocked, "I lost a parent and grieved that loss dearly." Her husband nodded in agreement.

Then the obvious question, "Do you have respiratory problems?"

Another very surprised reply, "Why yes, I do."

The lung problems most likely resulted in excess mucus that accumulated in the lungs. She may have developed a taste for hot and spicy food, which can dry out the lungs.

"Do you like hot and spicy food?" I asked.

She was shocked. At that point her husband said, "Yes, she does, and I can't stand hot food."

I massaged and pressed the lump. She felt a little pain at first, then many tingly energy sensations going down her arm. She reported that her shoulder pain disappeared, showing how easily she could move her arm. We sat and talked for a while longer. They finished by saying they would see me later. Unfortunately, I never saw them again.

Locating the Lg.1 acupoint is not always easy, but when you find it you will know it by the response. It is best to position yourself above and to the side of your partner. Massage the muscles (pectoralis major) above the breast. Massaging the area first, while you notice the muscles and bones, will aid in finding this important, energy-filled acupoint. Prepare the area by rubbing *(AN)* with finger circles on the upper part of the chest above the breast and below the collarbone (clavicle). To help in locating Lg.1, first find the locator acupoint, Lg.2, near where the collarbone meets the shoulder bones.

Lg.2 is in a notch beneath the collarbone and inside the shoulder bones. There is what feels like a rounded bone (coracoid process) to the outside of this notch. After you find this notch, measure one body inch (寸 cun sounds like "tsoon") down and slightly toward the arm; move toward the outside of the body as you continue down and over a finger-shaped muscle. There you will find Lg.1.

Another way to find Lg.1 is by locating where two imaginary lines cross. One line is straight across the chest below the collarbones with Lg.1 at each end: this line passes just below the place where the collarbones connect to the breastbone. The other line follows the contour of the chest from Lg.2 down and toward the side of the chest. Lg.1 will be found as you move down about an

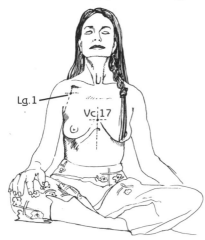

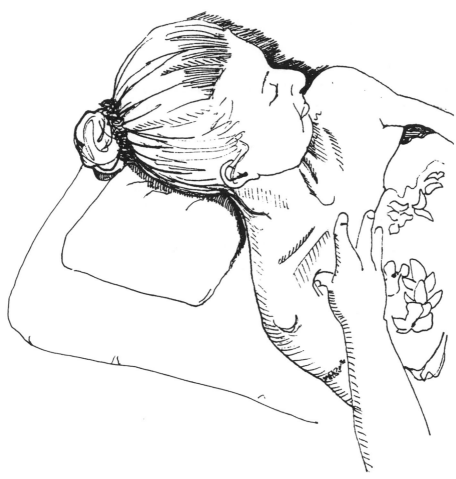

inch from Lg.2 in a separation between the muscles of the pectoralis major. Separate the muscles with your massage, then press *(MO)* in toward the heart. These lines cross where you will find a separation in a large muscle (pectoralis major).

NOTE: It is best to be positioned above and to the side of your partner's shoulder. Separate the muscles, then sink your thumb into a space between two ribs. The name ***Central Storehouse*** reminds you to direct the thumb toward the heart in the center of the chest when pressing this point. Remember, like all acupoints, Lg.1 is between the skin and the bone. First locate the point on the skin, then press toward the center of whatever part of the body, in this case the chest, on which the acupoint is found.

Hold for one to three breaths, depending on what it takes to get the energy moving. Lg.1 is a good energy point and an especially good release point. See if you can move energy all the way to the hand. If you cannot, that's all right. Get what you can, then after you are done pressing, rub the pectoralis muscles above the breast again. If you were not satisfied with the response, try pressing Lg.1 again. Then rub it out.

Do not be fooled by other sensitive acupoints in this area. They are not as powerful and do not radiate energy like Lg.1. Lg.1 is generally sore when the lungs are weak from chronic disease or when they are toxic from smoking cigarettes. It feels sore in a healthy person just before, during and after an upper respiratory infection. Many people feel an afterglow of increased circulation in the arm after the acupoint is released. This confirms the saying, "*Qi* energy commands blood."

This acupoint Lg.1 has its own peculiar *Deqi* sensation that is easy to provoke once you get a feel for it. The response may feel somewhat sharp, perhaps numb—like cutting off blood circulation—some say the feeling is 'heavy.' The arm may feel paralyzed, but while it may feel numb, it does not get cold and the arm moves easily, so it is not a true paralysis. In fact, stimulating this acupoint can increase circulation to the arm. This feeling of numbness is a common energy sensation. Your partner may feel it radiate to the little or index finger.

Move to the other side of the body, then rub the pectoralis muscle above the breast and below the collarbone (clavicle). Loosen it up. Find the locator point, Lg.2, where the collarbone and the shoulder bones meet. Press in and continue down a bit over the finger-shaped muscle that runs underneath the locator acupoint. Find Lg.1 where the muscle separates. Press Lg.1, hold it for one, two or three breaths. After the *Qi* moves, massage again, rubbing out the pectoralis and upper chest muscles.

Key concepts to remember about Lg.1:
- Location: On the chest one thumb width below the midpoint on the collarbone in a muscle separation, between ribs
- To find: Place hand on hip, move shoulder forward, the triangular hollow under the collarbone is the midpoint
- Deqi: Toward the hand and/or into the chest
- Use: Benefit the lungs. Improve the flow of surface energy circulation
- Pain: Chest, throat, shoulder, upper back
- Condition: Cough, cold symptoms, insomnia

攢竹

CUANSHU (ZANZHU)

Bushy Bamboo

UPPER SINUSES Bl.2

Bl.2 (Bladder 2) is named *CUANSHU*, which means **Bushy Bamboo,** and is nicknamed UPPER SINUSES because it brings sinus relief. The second *Pinyin* word *(ZANZHU)* is another way to pronounce the same Chinese character for bushy.

This acupoint can do much more, as I found out early in my massage career. When teaching at massage schools, the *Shiatzu* class I offered was popular with many massage therapists. They learned when they used energy points in their massage treatments for melting tension, instead of manually working out tension, they could work smarter, not harder—thus saving wear and tear on **their** bodies.

I worked in electronics, teaching *Shiatzu* in the evening for many years before I requested a fee for a *Shiatzu* massage. In 1980 the success of my classes encouraged me to retire from electronics and start a career in massage.

In the first year, an elderly woman came to see me. She wore a granny dress, bright colored running shoes, modest costume jewelry and almost no makeup. She said she had suffered from depression for years. I asked if she had sought medical help.

"Yes," she replied, "I've been to a psychologist. After a course of therapy he told me there was no psychological cause for my depression. It sounded to him like an energy problem. He suggested I needed energy work and that I seek an acupressure therapist."

Taking a closer look, I saw she appeared to be healthy. Tension showed in her face, but she smiled warmly. A determination to help this woman began to build within me. Something that caught my attention was her sneakers. It was not that she was wearing them that caught my attention, it was the colors of the running shoes—they did not match her dress.

I asked if she was on medication. She was not. Thinking the problem might be nutritional I inquired about her diet. (The shoes should have clued me into the fact that she was no ordinary little old lady.)

"I grow my own sprouts in a quart jar by the window," she declared. She ate whole grains and juiced fruits and vegetables. I didn't ask for more detail. Perhaps it was inactivity.

"Do you get exercise?" I asked.

"I walk at least two miles a day and up to five miles on some days." (I remembered the running shoes.)

"Have you ever thought of doing volunteer work?" I asked.

"Yes," she replied, "I volunteered at a senior citizen's center for a few years but hanging around some of those old folks can really get depressing."

Failing to find that her life-style caused the depression, I decided to give her a standard twenty-eight point *Shiatzu* treatment. She relaxed, never complaining about any of the acupoints I pressed. She seemed perfectly healthy. Then I reached the point **Bushy Bamboo** (Bl.2). I was pressing both acupoints with my index fingers in the familiar rhythmic manner: pressing with firm pressure for a short time, followed by a short release. Press and release, press and release.

She opened her eyes, looked at me and asked, "What did you do?"

I replied, "What do you mean?"

130

She said, "It felt like you released a tight band that had been around my head for many years."

The rest of the massage was uneventful. She said she felt much better and no longer felt depressed. I recommended a few more treatments thinking that she would soon be depressed again, that it could not be that simple. After two more treatments her depression had not returned. I had grown to like working on her. She was refreshing. But it was time to see if the treatment would last. I asked her to come back for *Shiatzu* three months later and, to make sure, one year later. Her depression never returned.

The interesting thing about Bl.2 is that it is not usually used for depression. Treating symptoms in the usual manner is not always the solution. Here a blocked acupoint had caused a low-grade headache that the client had become accustomed to. Even low-grade pain will steal enough energy that a person can become depressed.

This acupoint is located in a notch at the edge of the eye socket, in the bony structure around the eye, called the orbit. You can feel it in the upper part of the orbit, in a notch under the ridge near the bushiest part of the eyebrow. Thus the name, **Bushy Bamboo.** There is another acupoint at the outer end of the eyebrows, which is called **Silky Bamboo** Th.23 (Triple Heater 23).

Bl.2 is an excellent acupoint for draining the upper sinuses and improving most eye problems. It will even help rejuvenate the tissue in the forehead to counteract wrinkling. So, it is a cosmetic acupoint.

This acupoint prefers *(MO)* to be pressed and released. Press and release repeatedly with a pumping movement so you can experience why the pumping movement is preferred. Try experimenting on yourself by pressing long and strong. Learn to press this acupoint by experimenting on yourself. Find the notch, then press up and inward. Press firmly, stroking *(TUI)* left and right until you locate the most sensitive point. If the pressure response continues to increase until it hurts and you have to stop; you have located the acupoint. The intense pressure pain is not necessary to get a response. With a partner, if you press too hard or long, your partner may not let you touch that acupoint again. Worse yet, your partner may not let you touch anywhere again.

CAUTION: Do not press long and strong. It's too painful. Press and release, press and release with a pumping action.

Key concepts to remember about Bl.2:

- Location: On the face in the bushy part of the eyebrow
- To find: Press up and into a notch in the bony orbit
- Deqi: Around the eye and/or into the upper sinuses, possibly toward the neck
- Use: Clear the upper sinuses. Improve vision
- Pain: Eye, upper sinuses, neck, headache, hemorrhoids
- Condition: Sinus problems, eyestrain, insomnia

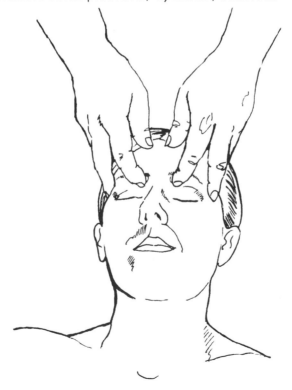

巨髎

JULIAO

Big Opening

LOWER SINUSES St.3

St.3 (Stomach 3) drains the lower sinuses and is used with UPPER SINUSES acupoint (Bl.2) for sinus relief. Many people with sinus congestion will discover this acupoint by themselves to get quick relief.

St.3 is located on either cheek, to the side of the nose. It is easy to find. Put your finger next to your nose at the level of the nostril, measure one finger away from the nostril, then rub toward the center of the head. As the Chinese name for this acupoint, **Big Opening,** implies, you will feel an indentation in the muscle. You may need to press around in the area to locate this acupoint accurately. If you have difficulty,

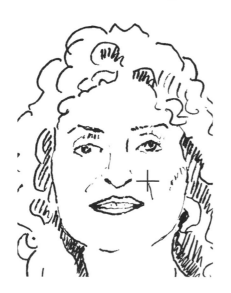

feel for the thickest part of the tissue, then move down a little pressing *(MO)* slightly upward. You may feel sensations in the gums and teeth, and into the sinus cavity.

For LOWER SINUSES (St.3) use the smaller fingers to do the pressing. The thumbs do not work at all. Index or little fingers will work best depending on the size of your partner's face.

Key concepts to remember about St.3:

- Location: On the face one finger to the side of the nose at the level of the base of the nose
- To find: Feel for an indentation in the bone
- Deqi: Into the teeth and/or lower sinuses
- Use: Clear the lower sinuses
- Pain: Lower sinuses, nose, teeth, lips, legs
- Condition: Sinus problems, swollen feet, facial paralysis

百會

BAIHUI

Many Gathering

STOP HEADACHE GV.20

The Chinese name for Gv.20 (Governing Vessel 20) is **Many Gathering.** It is nicknamed the STOP HEADACHE (including hangovers) acupoint. It is thought that this is where the energy enters or leaves the skull. It has also been referred to as the HEMORRHOID acupoint. The location near the twirl of hair on the top of the head, suggests the lines of force at the ends of a magnet—one pole at the top of the head and the bottom pole near the anus. The 'top-bottom method' of treating distant acupoints refers to the fact that we should work on the opposite end of the *meridian* to treat the disorder, thus Gv.20 benefits headaches and hemorrhoids.

This acupoint is associated with the brain. Gv.20 and Gv.16 are classified as *Sea of Marrow* acupoints. The Chinese term *marrow* can be translated as 'bone medulla.' The 'marrow' in ancient Chinese thought was the greasy substance located in the middle of bones, which is why the brain and spine, being grey and white greasy substances, are called marrow. The ancient Chinese healing masters noted that the marrow and the brain are both surrounded by bone. *Sea of Marrow* acupoints are associated with the grey matter of the brain. There are other marrow acupoints associated with the yellow and red marrow in the bone used to nourish the blood.

Gv.20 is found in the area of the vertex (the top) of the skull where the sutures all come together. After you have de-

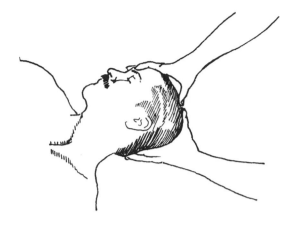

veloped a feel for the top of the skull, you do not have to measure. Until then, turn the head to the side to find the acupoint by placing a finger one body inch above the eyebrows and another finger at Gv.15 (at the base of the skull on midline in hollow between the uppermost neck vertebra and the skull). Find the midpoint between these two fingers, along the centerline of the skull, where you will find Gv.20.

Another way of locating this acupoint is with your partner lying face up. Put your hands parallel to the ground next to your partner's ears, reach with your thumbs across to the vertex of the head and press *(MO)*. Finish with scalp massage; fingertip stroking *(TUI)* of the scalp feels great.

Key concepts to remember about Gv.20:

- Location: On the midline of the scalp halfway between the base of the skull and a point one finger above the level of the eyebrows
- To find: Place a thumb one finger above the level of the eyebrows and the other at the base of the skull and reach for the scalp midpoint
- Deqi: Local
- Use: Improve mental clarity and memory
- Pain: Hemorrhoids, head (especially the top of the head, migraine)
- Condition: Stroke, shock, hypertension, dizziness

風池

FENGCHI

Wind Pond

Clear Senses Gb.20

To understand **Wind Pond,** the Chinese name for Gb.20 (Gallbladder 20), it's important to know the implications of the term *wind*. It refers to many symptoms and diseases that seem unconnected, yet it has much in common with the wind that moves leaves and blows trees down. Consider what you know about wind. The wind moves, yet it cannot be seen, however you can see its effect on things. It can be gentle or violent. It comes and goes unpredictably. Wind is commonly associated with the springtime; we say 'March winds' are good for flying kites. On the other hand, great winds bring destruction.

Have you ever wondered why North America has hurricanes while Asia has typhoons? In late summer, wind and rainstorms move westward across the oceans bringing much needed rain. When these storms are large and strike land, massive destruction takes place. The southern Chinese call these huge storms 太風, which means *great wind*. The northern Chinese pronounce 太風 'Tai fung'; in the south they pronounce the same characters 'Tai foong.' *Taifeng* (太

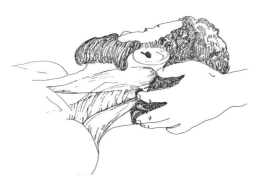

137

風) is the root of our word typhoon. Wind comes in many 'flavors:' it can be warm or cold, moist or dry. Hot dry winds that affect people emotionally are sometimes called 'devil winds.'

The *wind* attacks people like a storm. *External wind* disease attacks the outer body by starting near the surface and, unless it is stopped by the immune system, it penetrates deeper. For example, when a cold enters the mucus membranes of the nose or throat, it may then penetrate into the lungs where it can spread to other organs. *Internal wind* begins in the liver, blowing upward causing dizziness, muscle spasm or paralysis. It can hit deep in the brain, as in the case of stroke. *Wind* symptoms include spasms, weakness or twitching. They also include weather-related diseases like colds and flu. *Wind* diseases come and go like the wind (episodic). The term *Pond* reminds the practitioner that the acupoint is in a shallow depression where *wind* can accumulate.

Gb.20 is used when colds or flu attack. We say "avoid a draft" because the cold air on the skin can cause a headache, a cold or a stiff neck. The Chinese say a headache not associated with disease is called a *headwind*. Two types of brain injuries are associated with *wind*, one *internal* and one *external*. The *external* kind of extreme *wind heat* is called a *penetrating wind*, which we call sunstroke. An *internal* kind is caused by the *liver fire rising;* the Chinese also refer to this as *internal wind*. We simply call it a stroke. Dizziness and strokes can come and go like the wind.

This acupoint, when sore, indicates swelling and congestion in the head. Symptoms include nasal congestion, congestion in the eyes and headaches due to swelling, congestion and obstruction. Pressing Gb.20 acts to clear the head, including nasal passages, eyes and brain.

Locate Gb.20 at the base of the skull, three fingers to the side of the back midline, between two muscles. Find the muscle that attaches to the side of the skull, under and be-

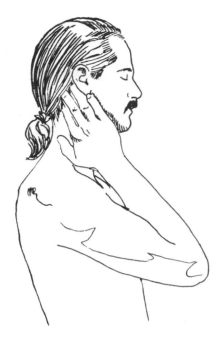

hind the ear. That muscle is called the sternocleidomastoid. Gb.20 is just behind it. When pressing *(MO)* this acupoint, make sure to direct your fingers up underneath the skull so that pressure is directed towards the eyes or the forehead. Always massage after pressing each acupoint. When Gb.20 is pressed, one may feel a sensation at the side of the head around the ear, eye or jaw. The sensation may end at the outer corner of the eye.

Key concepts to remember about Gb.20:

- Location: At the base of the skull about three fingers to the side of the midline
- To find: Press in a hollow under the skull where the muscles are the thinnest
- Deqi: Anywhere in the head, neck or shoulders (especially the eye and/or ear)
- Use: Improve hearing. Enhance vision
- Pain: Head, throat, neck, back, headache, migraine, earache
- Condition: Cold symptoms, swollen and red eyes, stiff neck, dizziness, hypertension

肩井

JIANJING

Shoulder Well

SHOULDER RELEASE Gb.21

The nickname for Gb.21 (Gallbladder 21), SHOULDER RELEASE, means this acupoint will release tense shoulders. Gb.21 is easy to find and press from any position. This acupoint became the first my students learned, because it's easy to find and brings immediate benefits. A good teaching principle is "Success breeds success."

On the first day of class, my students were paired off with the partner receiving in front of the partner giving the massage. Shoulders were squeezed using the pinching movement *(NA)*. The receiving partner's job was to give feedback on how it felt. Before long the room was buzzing with suggestions to pinch harder, pinch lighter or move a little this way or move that way. Soon, the sound of "Ahhh, that's great," was heard. It did not take long for the person receiving to figure out that, to get a good treatment, positive feedback is as important as corrective feedback.

My students had to find someone to help them with their homework. They soon discovered a positive side effect to asking friends to help: they all volunteered. Finding new friends to volunteer with homework became as easy as finding Gb.21.

There are also advantages to rubbing shoulders at work. One advantage is that relations between departments run more smoothly. The first time I went to the drafting department with drawings to be modified, I was directed to see the supervisor. He showed me a stack of jobs in his in-basket, which meant it would be a week before I would see my project completed. He informed me that this was the typical turnaround time.

After the draftsman had the drawings, I stopped by to check the project. I saw the draftsman bent over his table erasing and redrawing. I gave a couple of squeezes to his shoulders. He made a low sound of approval, so I pinched his shoulders firmly for a few minutes. A friendship started that continued for years. The massage I gave that draftsman did not go unnoticed by the other draftsmen. After that, instead of projects taking a week to be noticed, I got an immediate response. Taking projects through the door of the drafting department often prompted conversations and piqued interest in helping me with my projects as well as opportunities for me to rub some more shoulders.

The cooperation I received from the drafting department brings to mind something the cat said in the movie *The Cat from Outer Space,* "On my planet we have a saying: 'I'll rub your fur, if you'll rub mine.'"

Tension blocks the flow of *Qi* energy. Rub out tension, so life-giving *Qi* energy flows. As its name implies, **Shoulder Well** (Gb.21) is a source of life-giving *Qi* energy for the upper body, much as a well would be life-giving where water cannot be found on the land's surface. Also, when the tension is great, you will have to dig for this acupoint, just as a well must be dug to find water. The more tension in the shoulders, the less blood and *Qi* flows in the upper body. Gb.21 is nicknamed the SHOULDER RELEASE because it is an excellent acupoint for obtaining a release of tension in the shoulders so that energy flows.

It is easiest to locate Gb.21 on yourself, but first, notice how you feel, especially your neck, both shoulders, both arms and the sides of your chest (where the *Gallbladder meridian* flows). Now reach across your chest and place your right hand on your left shoulder near the neck. Hold your

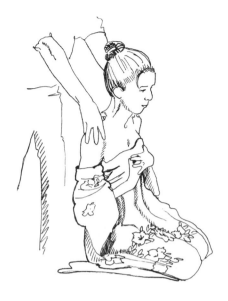

hand in the cupped position—the position used for rubbing *(AN)*. Make circles with your fingertips noticing how it feels as you massage the back muscles. Now keep the hand cupped while you stroke *(TUI)* your back and shoulder muscles (make sure the movement comes from your elbow) up and over the shoulder by pulling down with your right arm. Move your elbow down and to the right side. Stroke the shoulders firmly to push old stagnant energy out, making room for new energy. As you stroke your trapezius (a large muscle that covers the crest of the shoulder) notice that Gb.21 is the most sensitive spot under your second or third finger. This spot is most noticeable as you stroke across the shoulder from back to front.

How do you feel? How does your left shoulder, arm and side feel? If you feel much better from rubbing your right shoulders when you found Gb.21 on yourself, why not rub your left shoulder? Or better yet, ask a friend to rub your shoulders.

You can easily press *(MO)* Gb.21 on a partner in different positions: sitting up, lying on the back, or on the stomach. Locate this acupoint one body inch (about the width of your thumb) from the neck, where the shoulder and neck meet in the forward edge of the trapezius. It covers the shoulder completely toward the back, but it does not extend forward. On the front of most people, you can observe a triangular indentation above the collarbone (clavicle) and below the trapezius. Find the forward edge of the trapezius moving back about the width of your finger. You will be just on the crest, the high point, of the shoulder. Now find the point a

142

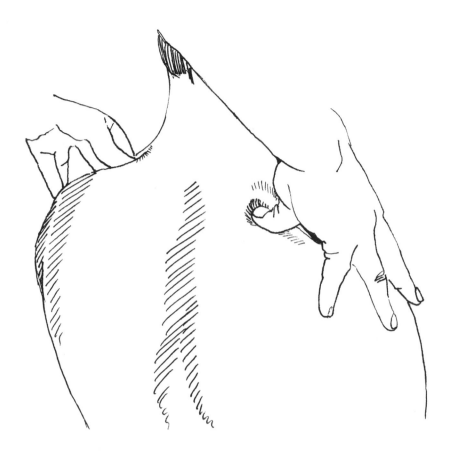

width of a thumb from the neck and press down (toward the center of the body) toward the feet.

To find the energy at **Shoulder Well** you may have to dig for it.

Some people feel sensations up to the ears where the energy flows along the *meridian*. Many people feel energy going upward. Some people feel it going downward. When muscles are locked up, tight and tense, the energy does not flow. Work slowly. Warm up the area before you press. Do some pinching on your partner, which is one of the nicest techniques to loosen the shoulders.

With your partner lying face down, place your hand on the shoulder while you press Gb.21. This will help to release the neck. Then pinch the shoulders again to see if they are loose. Gb.21 may be pressed again; it depends upon the individual you are working on. If your partner is not particularly tight in the neck and shoulders, you may want to press Gb.21 only once.

Key concepts to remember about Gb.21:
- Location: On the uppermost part of the shoulder along the ridge, one finger width from the neck toward the arm
- To find: Place thumbs on the crest of the shoulders near the neck and press toward the feet
- Deqi: Anywhere (especially the arms, head and/or back)
- Use: Relax the neck and shoulders. Move things downward.
- Pain: Shoulder, neck, back (especially headache due to neck tension, labor pain)
- Condition: Difficult childbirth, insufficient milk flow

天柱

TIANZHU

Heavenly Pillar

Nᴇᴄᴋ Rᴇʟᴇᴀsᴇ Bl.10

The Chinese name for Bl.10 (Bladder 10) is ***Heavenly Pillar.*** Its nickname is Nᴇᴄᴋ Rᴇʟᴇᴀsᴇ because the quickest way to release tension in the neck is to press Bl.10. As always,

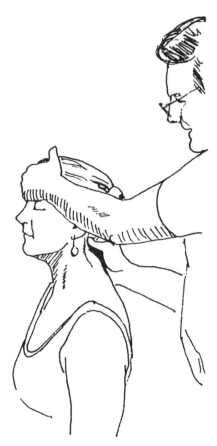

you need to be careful because massage makes some people uncomfortable. Look for what people communicate with body language. What do they do with their arms and legs? Are they protecting or opening? If you sense resistance, do not push it. It's always wise to get permission. Offer to rub out some tension. Listen to the tone of voice for permission to continue. It's not what they say, it's how they say it.

While working at an electronics firm, I was in the cafeteria on an early morning break. There were only a few people in the large room. I noticed the young woman from personnel communicating with her body language a clear message, "I have a headache." There are several ways this is indicated. She used her thumb and index finger to pinch her eyebrows together. She did not notice me walking over to her table until I asked, "Do you have a headache?"

She opened her eyes, looked at me and tilted her head in disbelief wondering, "How did you guess?" She revealed that she would wake up with headaches, usually lasting all morning, and sometimes all day. I familiarized her with acupressure; it did not take a car salesman to convince her to let me press some acupoints at the back of her neck. Five minutes later the headache reduced considerably. She called later to tell me her headache went away quickly after the mini-session in the cafeteria.

Months later, I was sitting at my desk planning my day when the phone rang. It was my friend with the morning headaches. Today it was particularly bad. "What are you doing on your morning break?" she asked.

I had nothing planned. "Meet me in the parking lot," I told her, "my van makes it easier to get the neck to release." She could lie down, I explained, while I pressed Neck Release, Bl.10, which would work wonders to relieve her morning headache. In the van there would be no distractions. The quiet would also contribute to a quick release. I pressed the acupoints, did a little neck massage and the tension melted away.

Looking up at me she smiled and said, "Thank you." That was payment enough for helping relieve her pain for another day.

Getting out of the van to return to work she turned to me beaming. Patting her disheveled hair, she gave me another big smile and said, "Wow, that was great. I feel so much better."

I thought nothing about the onlookers in the parking lot. Later my boss called me into his office saying there had been rumors that the secretary and I had been fooling around in the parking lot. After we talked it over, we had a good laugh. Fortunately, I had given him a few shoulder rubs and he knew me. Though I was eccentric, I could be trusted. He said, "Don't worry. If anyone else complains, I'll handle it. But I need your help. I'm having trouble getting some labels made in the print shop. Do you know someone in that department you could talk to?"

I replied, "There is a fellow who I helped after he hurt his arm playing baseball. I'm sure he could help us solve the bottleneck." We were back on schedule that day.

The acupoint Bl.10 is the tenth point on the *Bladder meridian*. The Chinese name, **Heavenly Pillar,** describes the location of the acupoint on the **heaven** side of the **pillar** that unites body and mind. The struggle between body and mind can produce tension at this acupoint. **Heavenly Pillar** is classified as a *Windows of Heaven* acupoint. This grouping of points promotes harmony between the body and mind.

Locate Bl.10 two fingers width to either side of the nape of the neck (Gv.15). Find Gv.15 underneath the skull in the center, above the upper-most vertebra. Press *(MO)* into the thickest part of the large neck muscles (trapezius) that attach to the skull. Feel for a separation in the muscles. Press into the separation, which may resemble a hole. Bl.10 is in the hole.

Position yourself at the head, with your partner lying face up. Feel for the acupoints on either side of the uppermost vertebra, place your index fingers on Bl.10, then lean back (see illustration on page 87). If the point is not too tender, you can lift the head off the mat a fraction of an inch. When your partner is sitting up, support the forehead with your passive hand while your active hand presses with the thumb and index fingers. Check to see that your passive hand is above the eyebrows. Positioning this hand over the front hairline is ideal. Then press your active hand in the direction of your supporting hand.

Bl.10 is a good point for release of tension in the neck. Often people will feel sensations flowing to the forehead while this acupoint is pressed. Press Bl.10 several times, rub *(AN)* and press, rub and press. Press and hold for one, two or three breaths, then massage again.

Key concepts to remember about Bl.10:

- Location: At the nape of the neck and two finger widths to the side of Gv.15
- To find: Press alongside the thick muscles into hollow under skull
- Deqi: Up toward the top of the head, forehead and eyes and/ or down toward the neck, back and feet
- Use: Clear the eyes and nose
- Pain: All types (especially in the head, neck, back, headache)
- Condition: Red and painful eyes, hypertension, stuffy nose, mental fatigue

Sixteen Acupoints for a Partner to Press

"There are three treasures in life: health, wealth and friends. Of these three treasures, health is the most important. Without health you cannot enjoy the other two."

"A little kindness at home is better than well wishes from afar."

—Ancient Chinese sayings

Although you can press your own points, the following points feel wonderful when pressed by a partner. If you have applied the knowledge in the preceding chapters, you have probably reduced tension and relieved pain in yourself and many people. Aha! Perhaps one of those people would like to practice finding points on you. Ahh. ...

"A friend is a gift you give yourself."

—Another Chinese saying

"Who pleasure gives, shall joy receive."

—Benjamin Franklin.

中脘

ZHONGWAN

Center Cavity

STOMACH Vc.12

Vc.12 (Vessel of Conception 12) is named the STOMACH point because of its location above the stomach cavity, in the abdomen. Vc.12 is classified as a *Fu System Gathering* acupoint.

In 1977, I enrolled my son in an alternative school called The Learning Farm. Some teachers lived on the farm. The farm had a goat, some chickens and a garden. The children helped with farm activities, attended classes and received individual tutoring. Parents were encouraged to participate. I offered to teach a *Shiatzu* class. Most of the teachers and a few older students joined the class. Interest was high on the first night. People were cheerful. They appeared to enjoy giving and receiving massage. After teaching Vc.12, the STOMACH point, I noticed one person after another getting up and leaving. Twenty minutes later, I was left with two of the twelve people in the class.

"What's going on here?" I asked. I was beginning to feel funny talking to only two people, wondering when the next person would leave.

One person still in the room laughed, "Oh, it isn't you, it's the cook."

A new cook, who favored hearty, heavy meals had many residents complaining of constipation. The STOMACH point (Vc.12) was the cure. Besides disrupting the class, this "cure" also created another problem. This was a farm with limited

150

toilet facilities. Some people could not wait and had to go outside in the bushes.

The name of Vc.12 is *Center Tube* or *Mid-cavity*, meaning the tube for food that runs through the center of the body. This acupoint is located near the center of the body's cavity where the internal organs are found. It is located on the abdomen above the center of the stomach. ZHONGWAN is a way of saying the pit of the stomach. Rarely painful, Vc.12 improves digestion by strengthening the stomach. Pain at this acupoint indicates the stomach, pancreas, or the entire digestive system in general has problems. Some people may feel energy radiate from this acupoint.

The STOMACH point also functions as the *Stomach Alarm* when it feels unusually tender to pressure. When something is seriously wrong with the stomach or pancreas, Vc.12 can-

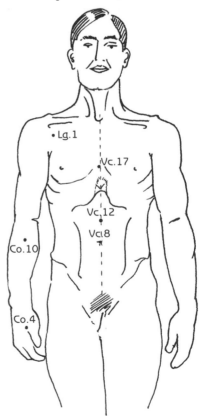

not be pressed even with light pressure for thirty seconds without causing distress. This same acupoint can be used therapeutically to benefit gastrointestinal disorders.

The STOMACH point, Vc.12, is located on the front midline near the middle of the trunk, the twelfth of twenty-four acupoints on the *Vessel of Conception*. When locating Vc.12, first find the navel (Vc.8), then (Vc.16) the bottom of the breastbone (sternum). Vc.16 is where the lower edge of the ribs meets the bottom of the breastbone (where the xiphoid process, a bone shaped like a triangle pointing down, attaches). Most students confuse the bottom of the breastbone with the bottom of the pointed bone (when it is deep, it cannot be found on everyone). Feel with your fingers for the rounded bottom of the sternum, not the pointed bottom of the xiphoid process. Vc.12 is located four body inches up from the navel and four body inches down from Vc.16, or halfway between the navel and the bottom of the sternum.

Rub *(AN)* the abdomen for a few minutes, then focus your massage above the navel. Locate the STOMACH point and hold for one to three breaths, remembering to avoid pressing *(MO)* on a pulsing object in the abdomen (the abdominal aorta). If you feel it pulsing directly under your thumb, move to the side. If you feel a pulsing in the area around your thumb, that is okay, just do not press directly on the artery.

Key concepts to remember about Vc.12:
- CAUTION: Do not press on a pulsing artery in the abdomen
- Location: In the pit of the stomach, on the midline halfway from the bottom edge of the breastbone (Vc.16) to the navel (Vc.8)
- Deqi: Upper abdomen and chest
- Use: Regulate vital energy. Detect difficulties with and improve digestion
- Pain: Abdomen, chest, stomachache
- Condition: All digestive disorders, nausea, mental stress, diarrhea, constipation

膻中

DANZHONG (SHANZHONG)

Chest Center

EMOTION OCEAN Vc.17

Vc.17 (Vessel of Conception 17) received the nickname EMOTION OCEAN from the observation that this acupoint is sore on people who tend to be emotional. The two-character word for the Chinese name has the image **Chest Center**. It is classified as an *upper energy point*, having to do with respiration. Vc.17 is also classified as a *Qi system gathering* acupoint. The two *Pinyin* words *DAN* and *SHAN* are two variations of pronunciation for the same ancient Chinese character for chest. This character is not used in modern Chinese.

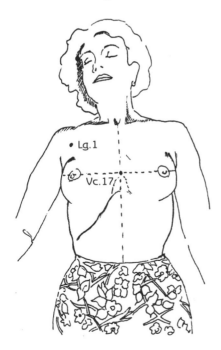

A system of therapy called the triple heater is part of Chinese medicine. There are upper, middle and lower heaters. Each heater represents a group of body functions necessary to sustain life's fire. The upper heater at Vc.17 is associated with circulation and respiration. The middle heater at Vc.12, discussed previously, is associated with digestion and assimilation. The lower heater at Vc.7 (one half inch above Vc.6) is associated with elimination—a combination of lower GI tract and urinary system.

Vc.17 is generally sore on more women than men. It has been said women tend to rely on their emotions and feelings more than men. Most men are not sore when this point is pressed, while more than fifty percent of women are sore. The Emotion Ocean (Vc.17) has a calming effect on the emotions.

Vc.17 is on the sternum (breastbone) in the middle of the chest. Located on the midline of the breastbone at the level of the nipples, it is in a hollow, one body inch up from the bottom of the sternum designated Vc.16 (see Vc.12 on page 150 for locating Vc.16). Another clue for locating this acupoint: on some people the flesh is thicker above and thinner below the point.

Key concepts to remember about Vc.17:
- Location: On the front midline at the level of the nipples
- To find: Press between the breasts one thumb width above the bottom of the breastbone
- Deqi: Chest, breasts
- Use: Calm emotional energy. Improve respiration. Regulate vital energy
- Pain: Chest, heart, breast, emotional
- Condition: Asthma, high blood pressure, insufficient milk flow, cough

啞門

YAMEN

Mutism Door

PRESSURE RELIEF GV.15

The Chinese name for Gv.15 (Governing Vessel 15) is **Mutism Door.** As the name implies, acupuncturists use this acupoint to treat mutism. The Chinese report success in treating children who have failed to speak. The term *door* used here implies that the acupoint works only one way, just as a door swings only one way, either in or out. Gates swing both ways. That means this point is not sore when someone is mute, but the point can be used to treat mutism. The nickname, PRESSURE RELIEF, indicates its more common usage. Gv.15 is good for stopping pain in the head. It can release pressure in the head, relieving stress headaches, sinus congestion and the pressure behind a nosebleed.

Every *Shiatzu* class I've taught has been special in some way. Not only have my students taught me many lessons, but I have also developed many wonderful friendships. One class experience brings a smile to my face to this day. It also began a friendship and business relationship that lasted many years. It all started while I was teaching the many uses of Gv.15. When I remarked that you can stop a nosebleed by jiggling the hairs at this acupoint located at the nape of the neck, one of the students at the back of the room started giggling. The giggle turned into a laugh that could not be ignored.

"What is so funny?" I inquired of the disruptive student.

155

"I've never heard anything so silly," she replied. I encouraged her to tell me more. "I'm a nurse for the local schools and children have nosebleeds frequently. At least once a week, I have to help an upset child relieve a bleeding nose. Often, blood gets all over their clothes. With all my training, I've never heard anything like what you're suggesting."

"Well, that's great," I replied, "perhaps by our next session, or certainly by the end of the class, you can report on the effectiveness of this technique." She gladly agreed.

The next week I asked the nurse if she had had an opportunity to try the technique for nosebleeds. Still a bit skeptical, she replied, "Once. And yes, it did work. However, it could have been a coincidence."

"Well then, will you keep a record and report to the class on the last day?" I asked. She agreed. On the last night of the class, I asked for her report. Something had changed in her attitude. She eagerly told the class that seven out of ten times the nosebleeds stopped instantly, and twice, it only took fifteen seconds to stop the flow of blood. She then related how one day she received a call from a distressed teacher at a distant school.

"You have to help me," the frantic caller demanded, "there is a boy whose nose is bleeding all over him and we cannot stop it. We cannot find ice and no one knows what to do."

Keeping her cool and thinking fast, the school nurse responded: "Okay, but do exactly as I say and don't ask any questions. First, distract the boy by telling him you want to look at his nose. Then, as he looks up, reach around and jiggle the hairs at the nape of his neck."

Silence. "Do you understand me?" the nurse asked.

"Yes, but ..."

"Just do it."

After a while the teacher returned to the phone and asked, "What happened?"

The nurse replied, "You tell me what happened."

"Well, I did as you instructed and the bleeding stopped instantly. But what happened?" the bewildered teacher asked.

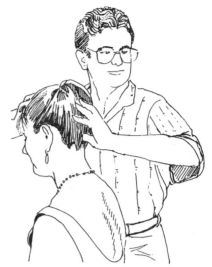

The nurse explained that it was an acupressure point that, when stimulated, could stop a nosebleed. Although there is no logical explanation, it does work most of the time.

A year later the nurse told me how the class had changed her way of thinking. She wanted to quit her job and start helping people with a massage practice. She actually did and we shared an office for many years. Her practice was a natural extension of her nurse's training; she was very successful.

Finding Gv.15 is easy—located at the nape of the neck. Gv.15 is on the back midline, above the uppermost vertebra and below the skull. A hollow forms when the head is tipped back slightly. Press *(MO)* this acupoint while your partner is lying on the back, side, or front, or even while your partner is sitting up.

Key concepts to remember about Gv.15:

- Location: At base of skull on the back midline in the hollow between the uppermost neck vertebra and the skull
- To find on a partner: Place thumb on acupoint and free hand on forehead. Move head back to form a hollow between neck muscles. Rub and press thumb toward the other hand
- Deqi: Local, possibly to the forehead
- Use: Clear the senses and the mind
- Pain: Head, jaw, earache, headache
- Condition: Nosebleed (pull the hairs to stop), TMJ syndrome, colds and mental stress

風府

FENGFU

Wind Storehouse

MENTAL ENERGY Gv.16

The Chinese name for Gv.16 (Governing Vessel 16) is **Wind Storehouse**. The term *wind FENG* is discussed in depth in the section on Gb.20. The term *Storehouse (FU)* has also been translated as *Treasury*; the same character is used to name Lg.1 *ZONGFU* **Central Storehouse**, which indicates that Lg.1 is the main storehouse for *meridian* energy. The character *FU* is composed of three simple ideographs: a person, a hand and a building. The image of a person (人) and a hand holding something (寸), when placed side by side, forms the character *to give* (付). *To give* in building forms the image of a storehouse (府). When a wind disease invades the head, it accumulates at this point and pressing this point relieves symptoms similar in action to Gb.20.

Acupressure massage benefits stroke survivors. A stroke, like the wind, can happen suddenly. The person gradually recovers to some extent, depending on how severe the stroke. **Wind Storehouse** is a good acupoint to stimulate mental energies and to nourish the brain.

Gv.16 is classified as a *Sea of Marrow* point discussed in the section on Gv.20. Both Gv.20 and Gv.15 benefit the brain, which explains its benefits to those who have suffered from strokes.

Gv.16 is just above Gv.15 in a notch on the midline just below the occipital protuberance. When you feel your partner's head, you will see that there is a prominent bulge just above the base of the skull. Just below that bulge there is often a notch. Sometimes it is very obvious, sometimes less so. You have to feel around to find a subtle indentation—similar to a little crack. Press there to stimulate the point.

Key concepts to remember about Gv.16:

- Location: About a finger width above Gv.15 toward top of head
- To find: Press against the base of the skull, in a notch below the occipital bulge
- Deqi: Local, possibly toward the top of the head
- Use: Stimulate mental energies
- Pain: Head, neck, headache
- Condition: Common cold, dizziness, strokes, numbness in limbs, mental stress

印堂

YINTANG

Seal Chamber

BLISS S-3

S-3 (Special 3) is named *YINTANG*, which means **Seal Chamber** and is nicknamed the BLISS point. The S designation means special or extra acupoint and is used to describe acupoints not on *meridians*. The character *TANG* of *YINTANG* (S-3) means (1) the main room of a house, (2) a lecture hall and (3) the courtroom in a government building. *YIN* means (1) an official seal, (2) a stamp, (3) to print and (4) to stamp.

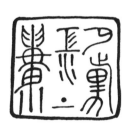 The character for *YIN* (印) has two parts, an image of the right hand (𠂇) and a stamp of authority (卩). A Chinese seal identifies an individual, taking the place of a signature or fingerprint. The king/ emperor issued seals to government officials to authenticate communication. Gold, silver or bronze seals were used to show the official's importance. Artists and prominent people created their own seals, while commoners used their fingerprints on official documents. The image of a hand pressing a seal suggests stamping. This image can also be seen as using the hand to stamp a fingerprint identifying the individual. The Chinese used seals to identify themselves on all correspondence, official documents and artwork. Seals took many shapes but never that of finger rings. In addition, sealing wax was never used, because the seals were not used to seal documents

160

but rather to identify the person who produced the correspondence or document.

Seals and Chinese characters have an association extending backward in time to the beginning of writing. Seals have been unearthed at the sight of the ancient Shang capital near Anyang. Chinese seals used red ink made with soybean oil and vermilion to stamp an image. Stamp pads were made from moxa (mugwort) wool or cotton batting. Today the oldest form of Chinese written characters are called 'seal characters' nicknamed 'tadpoles.' Only scholars of ancient Chinese writing understand them nowadays. Tradition says that Fuxi, the first legendary sage-king, invented the written pictograph. Some centuries later, the Yellow Sovereign (Huangdi) systematized Chinese writing. In the beginning, writing was only for matters of government and administration. Scribes were trained in official schools under the direction of a grand historian.

Around twenty-eight centuries ago (c. -800), Grand Historian Shi Zhou (sounds like "sure Joe") fixed the forms of all the characters and published a catalog. This script is called "Big Seal" characters (dazhuan sounds like "da chew+on). Scribes wrote with a type of fountain pen upon strips of bamboo or smooth wooden tablets before paper was invented. The large cumbersome instrument had a narrow bamboo tube with a wick, to regulate the flow of the ink from a reservoir above. Although slow, such an instrument traces lines in any direction either backward or forward, straight or curved. Therefore, seal character figures of every shape abound with the lines uniformly thick.

During the preceding Warring States period, Chinese writing had been adopted and adapted by various folks throughout China. The beauty of this system meant a clan or tribe could speak a different language and use the same written characters. The number of characters increased dramatically: besides new characters representing new ideas or things, errors crept in. Sometimes a primitive glyph as part of a composite character would be replaced by another sometimes-simpler glyph. The problem with this system was that these glyphs evolved into new characters and many were duplicates. Due to the lack of Zhou dynastic leadership, cultural studies and record keeping were neglected, bringing about the corruption of the language.

In the year -213, two important events occurred in the literary world of China that would be remembered to this day. First, the Qin emperor's chancellor, Li Si (sounds like "Lee zeh") published a new dictionary. Li Si's dictionary simplified and standardized the way thirty-three hundred characters were written. He also fixed a way of writing records kept by scholars. The new way of writing became the established form (font) for official government records, today known as "Small Seal" characters (xiaozhuan), a font used to write names and mottos when composing seals. Seal cutting, painting, calligraphy and poetry were the four arts traditionally acquired by anyone interested in becoming a scholar.

The second significant event in the literary world was the decree by the infamous Emperor Qin to destroy all classic books of literature. Many years later when the house in which Confucius had lived was torn down, old books written in ancient characters were discovered within the walls. At the sight of the big heads and the slender tails of the characters, the prince of Lu, who was not a learned man, exclaimed, "These are tadpoles!" That nickname for Chinese characters has stuck ever since.

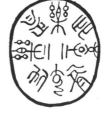

Shortly after Li Si published his dictionary, General Chengmiao, a Qin officer protecting the Chinese frontier, needed a fast effective way to communicate. He revolutionized writing by using a brush on strips of silk to write the characters. Drawn with a brush, rounded figures became squared, curved lines became angular, but this jerky writing was quicker. The small portable inexpensive brush soon replaced the awkward fountain pen device. Silk, and later paper, replaced expensive bulky wood and bamboo strips. Anyone could afford to write and read if they took the time to learn. Then an intellectual stream became a rushing river of knowledge as the brush became the current method of writing, while the "Small Seal" characters remained the classical writing used by scholars and employed on official seals.

The pituitary gland has a shape similar to a Chinese seal or stamp. Curiously, it is located in the bony chamber at the base of the brain with a narrow opening so small that it effectively seals the pituitary gland into this chamber. The nerves to the pituitary gland pass through this opening. This chemical-secreting gland, located in the center of the head,

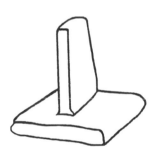 receives messages from the brain. These chemicals authorize the release of hormones that control certain bodily functions and human behaviors—just as the emperor's stamp authorized messages and commands sent to distant parts of the empire to control the functioning of the empire and human behavior. The acupoint **Seal Chamber** S-3 has a direct influence on and can be used to treat disorders of the pituitary gland. When this master gland establishes harmony between body and mind, a state of bliss may be at hand.

S-3 is located near the 'third eye.' It is interesting to note this point has been known since ancient times and it is physically on the Governing Vessel, however, it has not been classified as a Governing Vessel point. It is on the midline between the bushy part of the eyebrows, underneath the ridge of the forehead. This bony ridge between the eyes is where S-3 is found. S-3 is straight up the bridge of the nose at the base of the indentation below the eyebrow. With your index finger, point to a spot above your nose just below the line of the eyebrows, press *(MO)* up under the ridge. This is a good acupoint for calming the spirit. S-3 likes to be pressed firmly, long and strong.

Key concepts to remember about S-3:
- Location: Midway between the eyebrows under a bony ridge
- To find this sensitive spot: Press and rub up and down on the midline above the nose
- Deqi: Local sensation goes deep into the head, possibly toward the nose or upper sinuses
- Use: Calm the spirit. Relieve pain. Clear the nose
- Pain: Head, eye, nose, headache
- Condition: Hypertension, insomnia, hormone imbalance, mental and emotional stress

太陽

TAIYANG

Great Yang

AUDIO VISUAL S-9

S-9 (Special 9) is a common way to designate this non-*meridian* point, however a Chinese text would use the term *TAIYANG*, written in Chinese characters. *TAIYANG* is the Chinese word for the temple area on either side of the forehead above the zygomatic arch (the curved bone between the cheek and the ear). The temple-pulse can be felt by gentle but firm pressure of the fingers. A death sign can be observed in this area. As the light of spirit fades and death approaches, the temples sink, taking on a dark hue. The movie *The English Patient* demonstrates this in the death scene of the main character.

Great yang *(TAIYANG)* has many meanings besides the temple. It is an ancient word for the sun, as well as the name of the *Bladder* and *Small Intestine meridians* combined. The meridians of the body form a continuous loop of flowing energy, which means the last point on a *meridian* connects with the first point on the next *meridian*. The *Small Intestine meridian* of the Hand-*TAIYANG* runs from a point (Si.1) near the nail of the little finger, up the arm to a point (Si.19) in front of the ear. The *Bladder meridian* of the Foot-*TAIYANG* runs from a point (Bl.1) near the inner corner of the eye. From there it goes up and over the head and down the back to a point (Bl.67) near the nail on the little toe. The temple *(TAIYANG)* area is located between the end of the *Small In-*

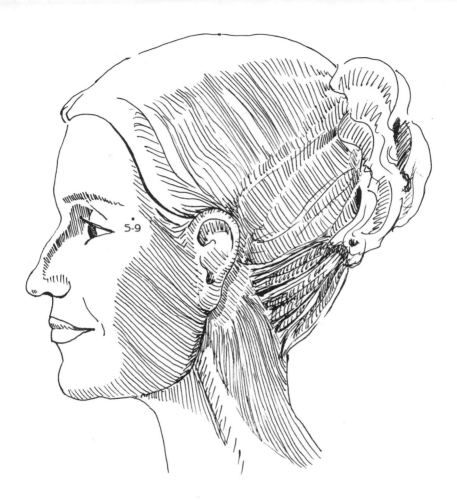

5-9

testine meridian near the ear and the beginning of the *Bladder meridian* near the inner corner of the eye.

The English word 'temple' is a curious word. Authorities disagree about the origin of the word temple. The *Dictionary of Word Origins* by Joseph T. Shipley suggests three meanings, (1) the body's tempo can be felt by the pulse and (2) the seasonable (opportune) spot hit by the enemy (page 290) or (3) Latin *tenuis* thus thin, the thin spot on the head (page 352).

Probably, the origin of the English word 'temple' is from the Latin *templum*, which derives from the ancient Proto-Indo-European root word *temp*, which means 'the arch of the sky.' *Temp* is the source of many other English words like template, tempo, temporary, contemporary, contemplate, temporal, temperance, temper, tempest, temperate, temperamental and temperature.

Ancient astronomers used an outstretched hand to measure the sky. Contemporary amateur astronomers do the same today. A star map was a template to measure temporal existence. An upright stick or a standing stone can be used to measure the time of day as the shadow moves from west to east, as on a sundial; when the length of the shadow is used to determine the time of year, it is called a gnomon. Standing stones were used as a template on earth to measure time in the sky. The ancient astronomer contemplated the sky to determine when seasonal temperature changes could be expected. Consequently, people could hunt animals when they migrated and gather plants when they were edible. Later, farmers used the tempo of the seasons to plant and harvest. Standing stones are sometimes referred to as 'sky calendars,' which became the first temples—

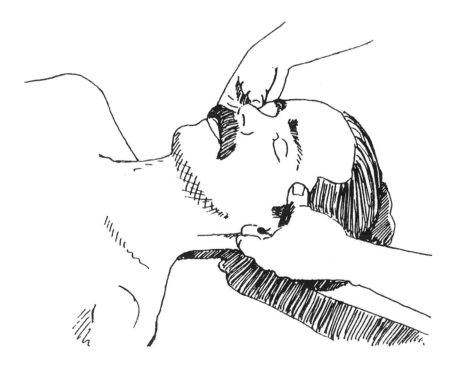

'heaven on earth observatories' where priests could communicate with the sky gods to predict the future.

Why did the Chinese call the sun *(TAIYANG)* the great yang? The Chinese have been observing, naming and classifying the stars since the Shang dynasty (-1766 to -1122) and perhaps earlier. Shang dynasty oracle bones mention many stars and constellations used in calendar making. Jade astronomical instruments have been found and dated to fifty-seven hundred years ago (c. -3700).

An ancient Chinese text describes the sun as great yang *(TAIYANG)* and the moon as great yin *(TAIYIN)*, whereas the stars are described as lesser yang and the planets as lesser yin. Earlier it was noted that yang is like fire and yin is like water. Yang fire radiates light; yin water reflects light. This ancient Chinese text correctly identifies the sun and the stars as sources of light and the moon and the planets as reflecting light (Needham, vol. III: 227).

I wondered whether the words temple and *TAIYANG* were related? Did one culture borrow the word from the other culture? And in which culture did the word originate? Linguists tell us that borrowed words must be similar in sound and meaning. A word meaning the area on the side of the head with additional meanings related to sky watching and time keeping may be a coincidence, but the similarity in sound is more than a coincidence. When comparing sounds, drop the vowels because they change easily, the consonants that remain must be similar. *TIAYANG* and *temp* are very close phonetically: t-ng and t-mp.

TAIYANG and *temp* are two ancient words from two cultures most authorities believe had very little or no contact before the opening of the Silk Road 2,130 years ago (-130). It was at this time the Han emperor tried to establish contact with the Great Yuezhi (Tocharian) tribe. They left northwestern China because the Turkic-speaking Huns from the northern grasslands killed their leader and made a drinking cup of his skull. These peace-loving people returned to their homeland in Russian Turkestan where they found a fertile valley to farm and raise their livestock, which included horses. The Han emperor wanted these fine, large horses, which he called 'heavenly horses.' He raised an army, conquering the entire area west to Bactria, the eastern most outpost of Alexander the Great's empire. He spent millions in gifts and bribes to maintain control and to be near the Tocharians, all to form an alliance against their common enemy, the Huns, but most importantly, to trade for their excellent horses.

In all probability the Caucasians who spoke Tocharian and the Chinese had contact. One culture adopted the word t-ng/t-mp into its language from the other, but which was it? Did the Chinese borrow it from the Caucasians or did the Caucasians borrow it from the Chinese? If it was borrowed after the opening of the Silk Road (-200), the Chinese borrowed the word from the Caucasians. If it was borrowed before, the Caucasians borrowed it from the Chinese, whose tradition of astronomy dated back thousands of years. Wouldn't it be nice if we could go back to the moment of cultural exchange that led to the sharing of this word? New discoveries often rekindle scientific controversies, answering questions as well as raising more questions.

A recent archeological find has shed light on the question of whether there was East/West contact at the dawn of Chinese civilization. Mummies with uniquely Caucasian features (redheaded, blonde and blue-eyed) were found in the Tarim Basin, a high desert in northwest China (west of the Yellow River and north of Tibet). Archaeologists dated these burials between twenty-four hundred to four thousand years ago (-2000 and -400). These mummies are thought to have belonged to a people called the Tocharians. An intriguing detail may answer the question about the origin of the word temple. A bearded man about fifty years old, who stood six foot six inches in life, was buried with his saddle around three thousand years ago (-1000). His mummified body was fully clothed with a rust-colored, two-piece tailored suit, bright red, yellow and blue striped felt leggings and deerskin boots. Most astonishing, there was painted on his temple, a bright yellow sun symbol spouting short and long rays. Did the three thousand-year-old man have a sun on his temple to represent the light of spirit, which glowed before the sinking and darkening of the death sign? Or did it mark him as an astrologer? The area above the zygomatic arch (the temple), could relate to the arch of the sky where the sun and stars are found. Questions still remain.

In light of this discovery, I believe around three thousand years ago (c. -1000) the Caucasians and the Chinese had a common word for the side of the head. As mentioned earlier, the Chinese classified the sun and moon as *TAIYANG* and *TAIYIN*. Therefore the Caucasians may have borrowed this word from the Chinese with their ancient star watching tradition. At this time the Chinese borrowed a cluster of words when they learned about chariots and weaving from the Caucasians. When an idea or an item is introduced into a culture linguists agree the word stays with it.

The acupoint is located in the deepest part of the temple area, below where the pulse is felt. It is one finger width posterior to the rear of the eye socket. Find that bony ridge to the side of the eye, lay one finger down and measure one finger over. When you press *(MO)* in deeply, you may feel a cord at the bottom of the hollow. Press on the cord for best results. Rub *(AN)* for a few minutes, then press, rub, and press the temples.

When *TAIYANG* is pressed on both sides simultaneously, the head feels a pleasant sensation, as if energy is passing between the fingertips. This will benefit the inner eye, inner ear and external ear. The nickname is Audio Visual or Sight and Sound because it benefits the eyes and ears. It is interesting to note that though this point has been known since ancient times, it has not been classified as a *meridian* point.

Body language for "I have a headache," is rubbing the temples. Circular massage feels good around the temples. It is the only place on the face where circular massage is beneficial. Generally circular massage relaxes and stretches the skin; this is not desirable on the face. The face muscles tighten in response to acupressure, which increases muscle tone producing a natural face-lift—circular massage on the face causes stretching and wrinkling.

Key concepts to remember about 5-9:
- Location: On the side of the face, a finger width from the side of the eye socket toward the ear, in a depression midway between eyebrow and hairline
- Deqi: Local and deep, when both are pressed at the same time the feeling is between the fingers
- Use: Improve inner ear. Benefit retinal functions
- Pain: Head, eye, ear, headache
- Condition: Dizziness, red swollen eyes

天宗

TIANZONG

Heavenly Ancestors

SCAPULA Si.11

The Chinese name for Si.11 (Small Intestine 11) is *TIANZONG*, which means **Heavenly Ancestors**. The name *TIANZONG* reminds one that the ancient Chinese used shoulder blades (Shang oracle bones) in a divination method of consulting with deceased ancestors and the Supreme Sovereign (Shangdi). The *TIANZONG* is also the name of a star in heaven.

Si.11, a good upper back release acupoint, is located on the back of the shoulder blade (scapula). It is easier to find if you remember it is the most sensitive acupoint in the middle of the shoulder blade. Locate Si.11 by rubbing *(AN)* your partner's upper back with finger circles. Notice where the triangular shaped shoulder blade is located on the back. It will help you in locating Si.11.

While massaging across the upper back from the shoulder toward the spine you may feel the spine of the scapula.

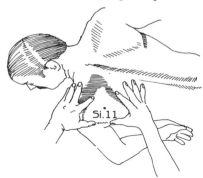

Notice the skin is attached to the bony process with muscles above and below. The spine of the scapula is the long curved bony process near the top of the shoulder blade. The Chinese called this the Great Wall. Look for the edge of the shoulder

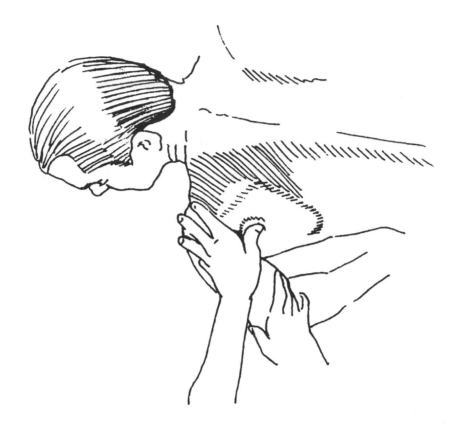

blade on the side toward you. Use fingertip movements to feel for the inner border of the shoulder blade, near the spine. Si.11 is in the middle of the triangular-shaped shoulder blade.

With your partner lying face down, the acupoint Si.11 can be located by measuring the distance from the bottom tip of the shoulder blade. First define the outline of the scapula by feeling for the bony ridge (spine of the scapula) across the top, then for the inner and outer borders. Si.11 is halfway between the two sides of the blade, two-thirds of the way up from the bottom tip toward the spine of the scapula. Besides using massage, there is another way to find the shoulder blade. Put your hand in the middle of the upper back to support it. Place your other hand beneath the front of the shoulder and lift up. This exposes the shoulder blade on almost everyone. Then find the two edges by imagining a line going right up the middle between the two edges. On this line you will find Si.11. Measure one-third of the way down from the spine of the scapula or two-thirds of the way up from the bottom tip. Now put the shoulder down and press *(MO)* the acupoint.

NOTE: Finding the Scapula acupoint that releases the upper back may be difficult, because this acupoint may be surrounded by other sensitive points that do not release muscle tension. The problem arises when areas of the shoulder blade around Si.11 are sore. These sore points may radiate that energy feeling *Deqi* into the arm but the upper back does not release. Because this acupoint can relax the upper back quicker than massage, keep trying, using massage and acupressure to release *Stagnant Qi* until the upper back relaxes. The problem of no energy response may simply mean more treatments are necessary. Interesting to note: if this acupoint is not sore when it is pressed, something is wrong. This is the only acupoint that is sore on healthy people when the energy is flowing.

Key concepts to remember about Si.11:
- Location: In the middle of the triangular shoulder blade
- Deqi: Toward the elbow, arm and hand, possibly toward the neck or deep into the chest
- Use: Reduce tension in the upper body
- Pain: Neck, shoulder, arm, chest
- Condition: Shoulder and arm numbness, asthma, cough, tender breasts

内關

NEIGUAN

Inner Gate

CIRCULATION Cs.6

The Chinese name for Cs.6 (Circulation 6) is ***Inner Gate.*** It helps with all types of *internal* problems, hence, the name. This acupoint benefits digestion, mental stress and heart problems. A great benefit is its ability to relieve nausea and pain in the pit of the stomach, deep within the body's trunk. The most common use of this acupoint today is stopping nausea. The best way to stop nausea is to press the acupoints on the right and left wrist at the same time. The effectiveness of pressing this acupoint has inspired the manufacture of wristbands that stop nausea, morning sickness or motion sickness. They are sold on cruise ships, in maternity shops and in health food stores.

The acupoint Cs.6 becomes sore when circulation and heart disorders are present, as the nickname CIRCULATION implies. Because this acupoint both benefits and warns of heart and circulation problems the energy is said to pivot both ways like a gate, as the name ***Inner Gate*** implies.

This acupoint affects the *XIN*. The Chinese character 心 *(XIN* sounds like "sheen") refers to both heart and mind. In ancient texts the character *XIN* refers to the pump in your chest and to mental functions. Many ancient people noticed that when thoughts of love or fear arose the heart beat faster and peaceful thoughts calmed the beating heart. Therefore, the idea of the heart as an organ of thought emerged. In the West we say, 'from the heart,' meaning the thought comes

175

from deep within. Use this acupoint to calm the mind and benefit the heart.

When someone in China has heart problems, it is recommended that circulation acupoints be used to benefit the heart. If this point is tender and you know you have heart problems, stroke *(TUI)* this point to get the benefits. There are many causes of angina. It could be simply a muscle cramp. It could be a small embolism. If the point fails to improve your condition, it may be time to get your heart checked.

The ancient healing masters noticed that if Cs.6 hurts and you rub it—it gets better. Then they observed that pain and disease on the **right side** can be benefitted by rubbing and pressing points on the **left side**. Further observations revealed that diseased *internal* organs cause acupoints on the body to become tender; they discovered that rubbing and pressing points on the arms and legs can heal *internal* organ diseases. When *Qi* energy exits, it warns that healing is going on by making an acupoint tender. By rubbing and pressing a point, *Qi* can be directed to heal distant parts of the body.

The characters *MEN* and *GUAN* are found in many acupoint names. The word *MEN* means a door, an entrance. The word *GUAN* means a gate, a barrier, as in a border crossing or a strategic pass. The secret to understanding these terms is knowing that a door swings one way; a gate swings both ways. At *Door (MEN* 門*)* acupoints, it is easy for *Qi* energy to enter, but it usually does not exit. At *Gate (GUAN* 關*)* points, it is easy for *Qi* to enter and to exit. What this means is that tenderness at **Mutism Door** (Gv.15) cannot be

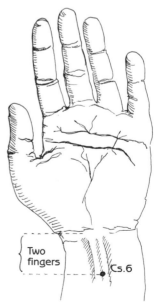

Two fingers

Cs.6

used to diagnose mutism, but it can open the voice on people who cannot speak. *Inner Gate* (Cs.6) works both ways: it can be used to evaluate *internal* disorders and treat *internal* disease.

The CIRCULATION point is located on the inside of the wrist where the tendons are easy to see. Measure two fingers toward the elbow crease from the wrist fold nearest the palm. The acupoint can be found between the tendons as you press *(MO)* deeply between the bones. When pressing Cs.6, you get more sensation when you press in firmly, angling slightly towards the thumb.

Key concepts to remember about Cs.6:
- Location: On the inside of the forearm 2.5 fingers from the wrist fold nearest the palm
- To find: Press midway between the two bones of the forearm and slightly toward the thumb
- Deqi: Toward the fingers and/or up the arm to the elbow, shoulders and chest
- Use: Improve heart functions
- Pain: All types (especially stomachache, chest, heart, arm, carpal tunnel syndrome)
- Condition: Nausea, insomnia, numbness, hiccough, heart problems

大杼

DAZHU

Big Shuttle (as in weaving)

CHIROPRACTIC RELEASE Bl.11

Bl.11 (Bladder 11) is classified as a *Skeletal System Gathering* acupoint, which explains how it received its nickname CHIROPRACTIC RELEASE. Pressing it releases tight back muscles, benefits the skeleton and speeds the healing of injured bones. Because of its proximity to the lungs, it is a good lung acupoint. This acupoint is also classified as a *Sea of Blood* acupoint. Now, of course, we know the marrow that makes red and white blood cells is in the bones. In fact, blood is created in the middle of the bones. So, here we have an acupoint that benefits the bones and the blood. All our red blood cells originate in the red marrow. It is inter-

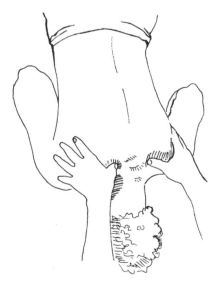

esting that even though this is where blood originates, the lowest circulation of blood is in the bones. *Blood* and *Qi* are required for health and healing. Increasing the circulation of *Qi* energy to the bones will benefit the *Blood*. Strengthening muscle and bone while tonifying *Blood* and *Qi* goes hand in hand when you press *(MO)* acupoint Bl.11.

Massage the upper back where a tee shirt collar crosses the inner *Bladder meridian*. Bl.11 is in the thickest part of the muscle on either side of the first thoracic vertebra (T1). To locate Bl.11, tip the head forward, then find the most prominent bone (dorsal process on the first thoracic vertebra) on the back where the neck and shoulders meet. Measure two fingers to either side of the tip of T1 and you will find Bl.11.

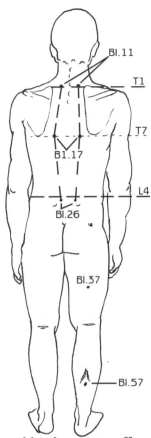

After your partner lies face down, position yourself at your partner's head so you can press Bl.11, holding both acupoints at the same time. Hold, hold, hold. Repeat this point several times during a massage session to reprogram the muscles to stay relaxed. The more the acupoints are pressed weekly, the more effective they become. Back muscles stay released for longer periods of time. Chiropractic treatments also release the upper back as the nickname implies.

Key concepts to remember about Bl.11:
- Location: On the upper back two fingers to the side of the back midline at the level of T1 vertebra
- Deqi: Local, deep into the chest
- Use: Speed healing of bone injuries. Benefit the immune system. Strengthen the back and neck
- Pain: Back, neck, shoulders, arms, headache, knees
- Condition: Back problems, posture, respiratory problems

膈俞

GESHU

Diaphragm Associated

GREAT BALANCE Bl.17

The Chinese name for Bl.17 (Bladder 17), *GESHU*, means *Diaphragm Shu or* **Diaphragm Associated.** Shu acupoints identify the body parts they are associated with. Other *SHU* acupoints are named after all the *internal* organs of traditional Oriental medicine. The word *GE* refers to the diaphragmatic muscle used in breathing. The acupoint is said to expand the chest, increasing *Qi* energy. It is classified as an important *Blood System Gathering* acupoint. This benefits *Spleenqi* and invigorates the circulation of *Blood. Blood* and *Qi* are benefitted by the GREAT BALANCE acupoint. Bl.17 feels sore when the body is out of balance. Weekly massage that includes pressing this point can restore balance.

Most Chinese names of acupoints consist of two written characters, therefore, more than seven hundred characters are used to make up the 365 names of the *meridian* acupoints. Many are used repeatedly. The character for *SHU, Associated,* is found in twenty-five names including: **Diaphragm Associated** Bl.17 and **Gate of Origin Associated** Bl.26. Nineteen *Associated* (*SHU* 俞) acupoints are on the *Bladder meridian* and six are on other *meridians*. The character for a *Door (MEN* 門) is found in twenty-two names including: **Abundant Door** Bl.37 and **Mute Door** Gv.15. The character for *Gate (GUAN* 關) is found in fourteen names including: **Gate of Origin Associated** Bl.26 and **Inner Gate** Cs.6. *Bone-opening (LIAO* 髎) is found in fourteen names including: **Big Opening** St.3. The character for *Center (ZHONG 中)* is found in twenty names including: **Center Cavity** Vc.12, **Chest Center** Vc.17 and **Central Storehouse** Lg.1. The image *Heaven (TIAN 天)* is found in sixteen names including: **Heavenly Ancestors** Si.11 and **Heavenly Pillar** Bl.10. The character representing *Yang (陽)* is found in eighteen names and *Yin (陰)* in fourteen names as in **Three Yin Crossing** Sp.6.

Bl.17 is two fingers to either side of the back midline at the level of the seventh thoracic vertebra (T7). T7 is level with

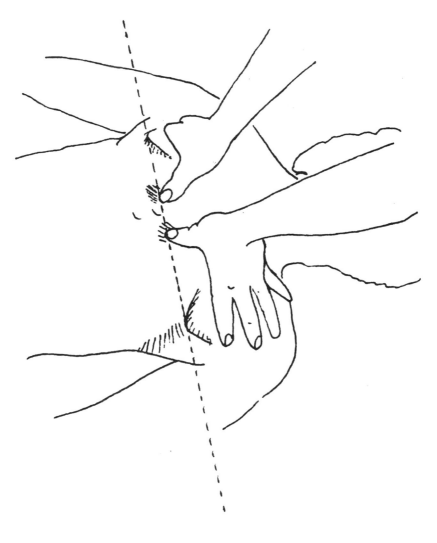

the bottom tip, or apex, of the shoulder blade (scapula). When a line is drawn between the bottom tips of the two shoulder blades it will cross the back at T7. Now measure two fingers to the side of the T7 vertebra. Tension can move the shoulder blades into the wrong position for measuring, or the shoulder blades may have different shapes or lengths. Occasionally you may have to count vertebrae to exactly locate this acupoint. Counting vertebrae is not always the easiest way to locate T7 and can result in missing the acupoint. Stroke *(TUI)* up and down the spinous muscles asking the person, "Is this sore?" If there is only one sore spot on the midback and it is not very sore, it is probably Bl.17. Using several methods to find this or any acupoint is the best way to locate an acupoint.

Key concepts to remember about Bl.17:
- Location: In the middle back two fingers to side of back midline, level with the lower tip of shoulder blade
- To find: Have arms at side, so shoulder blades are in normal position
- Deqi: Local, deep into the chest
- Use: Improve breathing capacity. Strengthen the back. Cleanse the blood
- Pain: All types (especially back, chest, heart, stomachache, skin)
- Condition: Hiccough, backache, digestion, fatigue

關元俞

GUANYUANSHU

Gate of Origin Associated

Baby Bl.26

The location of Bl.26 (Bladder 26), called *GUANYUAN-SHU*, on the back, is exactly opposite a point on the abdomen called *GUANYUAN* (Vc.4). Two characters make up the word *GUANYUAN*. (Again *GUAN* means *Gate*.) *YUAN* is a term that means first, primary, basic or fundamental. *YUANQI* is basic vital energy that is stored in the kidneys and delivers dynamic health.

The Baby point nickname is an apt one. The cervix of the uterus is the original 'gate' through which sperm enter the

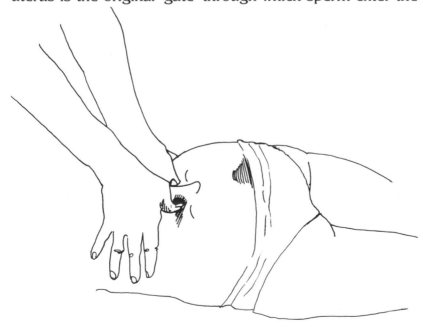

womb; through this gate the baby enters the world. Therefore, **Gate of Origin** is an appropriate name for an acupoint associated with the reproductive organs. This is an effective acupoint for women having menstrual problems and during the birthing process it opens the cervix. This acupoint benefits the male reproductive organs as well.

Locate Bl.26 on the low back in the thickest part of the back muscle, one finger width to either side of the fifth lumbar vertebra (L5). This acupoint is located below the beltline and above the large bone at the base of the spine (sacrum).

When your partner is laying face down, position yourself near the head placing your hands so that the fingertips reach around the sides to the crests of the hipbone (ilium). With your thumbs on Bl.26, press *(MO)* deep angling toward the feet. Most people enjoy having this point pressed, unless they have a problem. In that case, improve the circulation of *Qi* and *Blood* by massaging and pressing in the area of Bl.26.

Key concepts to remember about Bl.26:
- Location: In lower back two fingers to side of back midline, in a hollow above sacrum and below waistline
- To find on a partner: Place fingertips on hipbone at side and thumbs on back muscles. Press in toward feet
- Deqi: Local, may radiate into the hips and legs
- Use: Promote longevity. Improve the sexual function. Strengthen the back.
- Pain: All types (especially back, leg, abdomen)
- Condition: Indigestion, bladder infection, childbirth

環跳

HUANTIAO

Twist and Jump

JOINT POINT Gb.30

The Chinese name for Gb.30 (Gallbladder 30) is *HUAN-TIAO*, which means **Twist and Jump.** The name suggests that this acupoint benefits the rotator muscles in the hip, which are essential to our ability to jump and turn around. The nickname, JOINT POINT, reminds us that this point affects the hip joint.

This acupoint strengthens the lower back while alleviating pain in the legs, especially sciatica. This acupoint should be checked when there are problems in the torso and the leg. Press Gb.30 to release the back muscles. At this acupoint, the *Gallbladder* and *Bladder meridians* come together.

Gb.30 is located in the dimple of the buttocks. To locate this point, first find the large triangular bone at the base of the spine and between the buttocks (sacrum). Next find the most prominent bony process (hiatus of the sacrum) found where the tailbone attaches and curves inward. Next find the bony tip at the top of the thighbone (greater trochanter). Find the greater trochanter by pressing the fingers of your open flat hand against the side of the hip. To locate the bony process (greater trochanter), press the flat of your hand firmly while you rotate your partner's leg. The bone that moves under the skin is the greater trochanter. Gb.30 is on the side of the buttocks two-thirds of the way from the hiatus toward the greater trochanter.

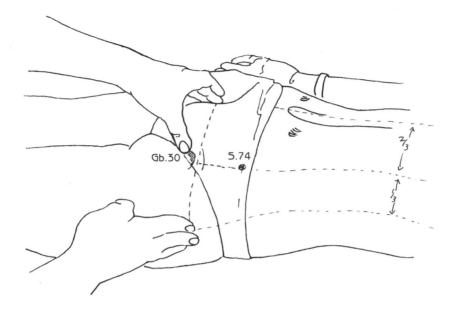

Gb.30   5.74

The secret to locating this point with your partner lying face down, is to use one hand to turn the leg so that the toes point inward, while the other hand rubs *(AN)* and strokes *(TUI)* the buttocks looking for a separation in the muscles. If your partner's toes are pointed outward, you may have difficulty pressing Gb.30.

Be careful with pressure *(MO)* on this acupoint, it might be tender. Prepare the buttock by using *Shiatzu* movements; pinching *(NA)*, finger circles, heel of hand and gentle thumb stroking. Good firm squeezes will often release the hip muscles, getting rid of old stagnant energy, which makes room for new fresh energy. Rub *(AN)* with your thumb making circles, push more muscles out of the way and rub again. If you work slowly and the point is not tender, you may be able to feel deeply into the hip joint. Press and hold Gb.30. It's like a 'window' into the hip; the muscles separate, allowing you to 'look' into the joint. After you have pressed Gb.30, rub it out.

Key concepts to remember about Gb.30:

- Location: Deep in the buttocks, two-thirds the distance from the base of the sacrum toward the greater trochanter (a prominent leg bone at the side of the hip, eight fingers below the hip bone)
- To find: Point toes inward, then press and rub gently. Press deeper only as tension eases and the muscles separate
- Deqi: Local, deep into hip, low back, genitals and/or down the leg, knee, foot
- Use: Clear the channels. Strengthen the back and legs
- Pain: Back, hip, leg, sciatica
- Condition: Back strain and stiffness, tired legs, stroke, numbness

跳躍

TIAOYUE

Leap

SCIATICA RELIEF S-74

The nickname for S-74 (Special 74), SCIATICA RELIEF, reveals the interesting fact that there are two types of sciatica: 'true' and 'false.' True sciatica means that the sciatic nerve is inflamed, causing a painful, often numb feeling in the leg. False sciatica is caused by muscle tension alone. When this point brings some relief, the indication is that regular treatments can bring complete relief using this and other therapeutic acupoints (see pages 206 and 226 in **Acupressure Therapy** for more acupoints). S-74 is a non-*meridian* acupoint with a name similar to Gb.30. *TIAOYUE* (S-74) means **Leap**. It will often benefit hip problems that **Twist and Jump** (Gb.30) fails to help.

S-74 is located in the buttock muscle four fingers toward

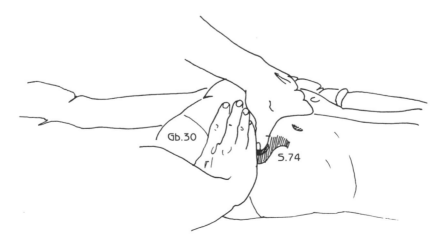

the head from Gb.30. Measure two hand spans between Gb.30 and the crest of the hipbone (ilium). Check that you are pressing on an imaginary line parallel to the back and side midlines. The acupoint is on that line four fingers below the crest of the hipbone. Often you will find a cigar shaped muscle right beneath S-74. Press *(MO)* and hold for one to three breaths.

Use pinching *(NA)*, finger circles, thumb stroking *(TUI)* and the heel of the hand *(AN)* to warm up the buttocks (gluteal muscle). Be careful. This acupoint can be tender on some people. If you feel it relax and release, your partner may feel the energy moving around in the body after rubbing it out.

The Chinese people enjoy traditional sayings passed down from ancient times. They also love humorous stories to make their point. One such story goes like this:

A scholar versed in ancient and modern literature but inexperienced in the ways of common folk was on a holiday. While on a walk during his first visit to the countryside, his path was blocked by an irrigation canal. He asked a farmer who was tilling a field nearby, "How can I get to the other side of this ditch?"

The farmer replied, "It's easy. Don't be afraid. Just jump over it."

He planted both feet firmly near the edge and jumped, but his efforts fell short. He found himself waist deep in the water. When the farmer came to drag him out of the ditch, he advised, "You shouldn't jump with your feet together."

The scholar replied, "The dictionary definition of jump means spring up with both feet together. Why didn't you tell me to leap? Leap means to push off with one foot while leading with the other. Then I could have crossed this ditch with ease."

The farmer replied, "I'm only an ignorant farmer I don't know the definitions of words, but I know how to cross a ditch."

Do not misunderstand the meaning of this story. It is not a diagnostic method to determine whether to use **Leap** (Gb.30) or **Twist and Jump** (S-74). If your partner has low back or hip pain, use both acupoints. This story illustrates in a humorous way that books may enlighten the mind but are no substitute for the practice of living. If you have read this book to this point and you have not found these acupoints on another person, take the leap now. A common Chinese saying advises, "Without experiencing a thing, one does not gain knowledge of it." Many people have back and hip pain. Rub and press the above acupoints along with **Gate of Origin Associated** (Bl.26 on page 123) and **Abundant Door** (Bl.37 on page 191). See if you can change suffering into a smile.

Key concepts to remember about S-74:
- Location: In the buttocks one-third the distance from the side midline toward the back midline, four fingers below the hip bone (iliac crest), four fingers above Gb.30
- To find: On a partner press on a finger shaped muscle
- Deqi: Down the leg, knee and foot and/or low back
- Use: Relax the buttocks
- Pain: Back, hip, leg, sciatica
- Condition: Sciatica, numbness, sexual dysfunction

殷門

YINMEN

Abundant Door

THIGH Bl.37

The Chinese name for Bl.37 (Bladder 37) is *YINMEN*, which means *Abundant Door.* A rear view of the thigh muscles resembles a swinging door. The release button, which unlocks tension in the thigh, is found near the back midline of the thigh. The word *MEN (Door)* is an acupuncture term which means a point may only work one way, namely to benefit, compared to *gate* points which telegraph tenderness when something is wrong. This acupoint need not be tender to bring great benefits in releasing and strengthening the thigh muscles. The character for *YIN* of *YINMEN* means very much, great, abundant, the center, or exactly.

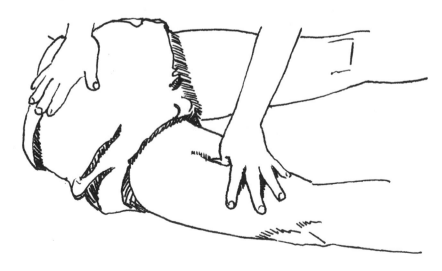

Bl.37 is located on the back midline of the thigh, halfway to a soft spot behind and above the knee (the popliteal fossa) from the crease where the thigh meets the buttocks (the gluteal fold). The secret to locating this point is to find the separation between the muscles on the back of the thigh. This becomes easier as the thigh relaxes. Prepare the thigh with firm squeezes using muscle pinching *(NA)* as well as finger circles *(AN)*, heel of hand and thumb stroking *(TUI)*. If the muscles remain tight, use more vigorous movements on the thighs. Once the thigh starts to soften up, look for where the muscles separate while you massage.

Now find locator acupoint Bl.36 near the center of the gluteal fold where the thigh meets the buttocks. It's a soft spot that can be pressed *(MO)* deeply. Bl.36 is at the top of this muscle separation. Now find the crease behind the knee, measuring three fingers up the leg, feeling for a soft spot above the back of the knee (popliteal fossa). Bl.37 is halfway between Bl.36 (the gluteal fold) and the popliteal fossa. Push into the back of the thigh where the muscles separate into two groups: left and right. Press and hold. It usually takes about three breaths to get a good release. You may even want to press it twice. Press and hold. When the thigh is large, you may want to use your elbow. After pressing the acupoint, massage out the released energy.

Key concepts to remember about Bl.37:
- Location: On back of thigh halfway between the soft spot above the knee and the buttock fold
- To find: Press into a natural division of the muscles
- Deqi: To the low back and/or knee, foot
- Use: Strengthen the legs
- Pain: Back, hip, leg, sciatica
- Condition: Stiffness and numbness of the leg

承山

CHENGSHAN

Support Mountain

Calf Bl.57

The Chinese name for Bl.57 (Bladder 57), *CHENGSHAN* means **Support Mountain.** The calf muscle (gastrocnemius) looks like a mound; the acupoint is at the base where the 'river' of energy comes out of the 'mountain.' I just call it the Calf acupoint. It is a whole-body muscle-release acupoint. It also helps to relieve constipation.

To locate Bl.57 on the back of the calf between the two heads of the calf muscles (gastrocnemius), measure along the back midline, midway between the tip of the external anklebone and the crease behind the knee. Place your fingertips at both locator points and stretch

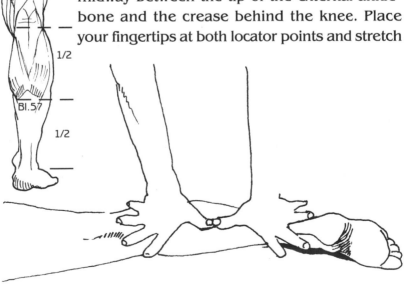

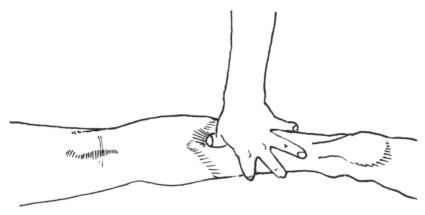

your hands so that your thumbs cross or try to meet at mid-point. Touch both anklebones at the same time with the fingertips of one hand, checking that you are at the bottom tip of the anklebone. If you are high on the anklebone, you will be measuring from the wrong place.

Use caution. Remember some people are very tender on the inside of the calf, so start out with a gentle pinch (NA) working into a stronger pinch. Be aware of any reaction, then gradually change to a faster movement. Use pinching as the technique of choice to massage the calf.

Thumb stroking (TUI) up the middle feels good to some people. Small circles (AN) made with the fingertips can help find where the muscles separate. Measure halfway between the external anklebone (the external malleolus) and the crease behind the knee (the popliteal crease) to find the acupoint.

Key concepts to remember about BI.57:
- Location: On back of the calf on the midline, halfway between the knee crease and external ankletip
- To find: Rub and press a point on a tendon where the belly of the muscle splits in two
- Deqi: Up or down the leg, possibly to the knee or hip
- Use: Relax all muscles. Improve bowel functions
- Pain: Back, legs, sciatica,
- Condition: Weak legs, constipation, hemorrhoids, muscle spasm

血海

XUEHAI

Blood Ocean

Sp.10

The name for Sp.10 (Spleen-Pancreas 10), ***Blood Ocean*** reminds us that this acupoint will nourish and detoxify the *Blood*. *Blood* disorders that can be benefitted include menstrual problems, anemia, or poor circulation. Pressing this acupoint is also indicated for skin problems such as itching and rashes, which are caused by toxic blood.

Sp.10 is located on the inside of the thigh, at a level two fingers above the kneecap. From the side of your partner, reach over the thigh with your fingertips feeling for a separation between the front muscle group (quadriceps) and rear muscle group (hamstrings). Finally, measure one finger width into the quadriceps muscle from the separation. Feel for a knot in the muscle tissue.

This acupoint may be difficult to locate because of painful muscles or ticklish legs. A gentle but firm massage will disperse the old stagnant energy in order to allow probing the ***Blood Ocean*** acupoint. Slowly squeeze the thigh above the kneecap, pinch *(NA)*, hold and release, pinch, hold and release. Many people are ticklish; they will only allow firm muscle pinching and acupressure *(MO)*. Sometimes a little stroking *(TUI)*, but nothing too vigorous, will be tolerated. Pinch the front of the thigh with a firm rhythmic squeeze and release before you try more vigorous pinching. Squeeze and release. Then, if you can massage more vigorously without getting an unwanted reaction, use alternate pinching and thumb stroking.

Key concepts to remember about Sp.10:

- Location: In the thigh, with leg straight (see below), two fingers above the kneecap on the inside of the thigh near the edge of a muscle (quadriceps)
- To find: On yourself sit with knee bent, place right palm on left knee. Find acupoint at tip of thumb inside thigh
- Deqi: Toward the knee and/or up the leg, possibly to the groin
- Use: Harmonize blood function. Regulate menstrual flow. Benefit the skin
- Pain: Menstrual, knee, legs, genital
- Condition: Menstrual problems, itching, rash, fever, knee pain

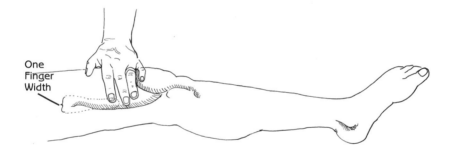

One Finger Width

A *Shiatzu* Session

In the *Shiatzu* session your knowledge and experience of the acupoints and movements come together. Knowledge of the movements and acupoints comprise the science of *Shiatzu*. Translating this knowledge into a successful session is the art of *Shiatzu*.

Preparations

Ask your partner to follow these suggestions prior to the *Shiatzu* session:

- Refrain from eating just before a session. Allow one hour for a light meal of fruits or vegetables to digest. Allow three hours for meat or a heavy meal to digest.
- Avoid strenuous physical activity for at least thirty minutes before a session.
- Avoid the use of pain-killing or psychoactive drugs for at least four hours before the session. When you are under the care of a physician, consult with him/her about reducing dosage and the advisability of acupressure massage.

Traditionally *Shiatzu* is performed on a person in a kimono. When learning to perform *Shiatzu*, the partner receiving can help by wearing as little as possible: loose cotton clothing, bathing suits or underwear. You may want to drape the body with sheets or towels for the sake of modesty. With experience you will be able to find the acupoints with ease, even when your partner is fully clothed. Keep a notebook and pencil at your side to note sensitive acupoints, signs and complaints. You may want to make notes in this book as well.

Precautions

If you **do not know** your partner's state of health, **ask**. *Shiatzu* is not designed to cure illness but to promote health. If your partner has a contagious disease or a broken bone, do not perform *Shiatzu*. If you reach a point during the session where you do not know what to do, the best rule is to **do nothing**.

Aside from illness, *Shiatzu* is not appropriate when a person has been drinking alcohol, has taken drugs, has eaten a large meal, or is extremely tired. For someone who is very hungry, offer a glass of juice before beginning the session.

Position

Kneel or sit beside your partner with your knees the space of a fist away from your partner's body. If your legs hurt, shift your position or do some quick *Shiatzu* on yourself. In most cases, muscle pinching *(NA)*, then pressing the release acupoints and finally stretching will improve circulation enabling you to sit comfortably.

Sitting beside your partner, face their body while extending your arms. Rest one hand on the abdomen and the other on their leg or upper chest.

Centering

By being centered, your *Shiatzu* induces balance and relaxation. Before beginning *Shiatzu*, take a few moments to center yourself as follows:

* Relax. Focus your attention on your abdomen *(Hara)*. Concentrate on your lower abdominal acupoint called the *Sea of Energy* (Vc.6) located below the navel. Sit upright and breathe out slowly.

- Expel your breath slowly and forcefully using your abdominal muscles.
- Let go of your focus in the *Hara* and focus your attention on your hands. Notice the palms in contact with your partner, see how they rise and fall with your partner's breathing.
- Synchronize your breathing with that of your partner. Breathing in and out with your partner will develop a rapport that facilitates *Shiatzu*.
- A moment later, let go of breath awareness and begin giving *Shiatzu*.

The Basics of a *Shiatzu* Routine

To perform the basic *Shiatzu* routine, work on one area at a time in the order described following these basics. In general, the routine proceeds as follows:

1. Begin with a light *Shiatzu* to evaluate the area, searching for sensitive acupoints. Work on the surface, using large circles, fast rhythm and light pressure.
2. The next time, if the signs are not contrary, give a moderate *Shiatzu*, using a moderate pressure.
3. If a sensitive acupoint is discovered, determine whether the pain is mild (annoying), uncomfortable (tiring), or distressing (miserable). Apply moderate pressure with the fingers. Ask your partner to judge the degree of pain experienced. Treat a sensitive acupoint by giving a light, slow *Shiatzu*. If pain is distressing and you do not know its cause, refer your partner to a doctor. **If the pain is uncomfortable do not work deeper.**
4. Desensitize an area before proceeding to a deep *Shiatzu*. You will soon develop the ability to sense the appropriate degree of pressure. Work no

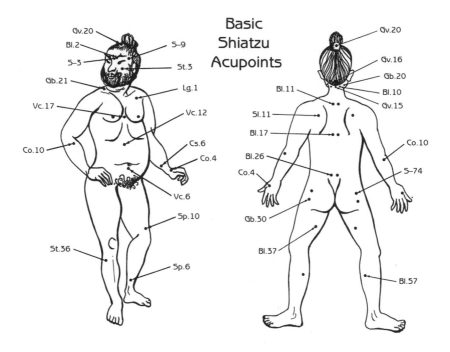

Basic Shiatzu Acupoints

deeper than the gray area between pleasure and pain. Breathe with your partner. Apply pressure to the acupoints in the area as you both exhale.

5. Finish the area with a light *Shiatzu,* leaving it with a good feeling of tingling, warm, glowing energy.

Occasionally students will find that after giving a *Shiatzu,* they feel drained of energy or they develop some of their partner's complaints, such as a stiff or sore arm. These responses on your part indicate that you need to spend more time centering yourself before beginning *Shiatzu.* Try reviewing this book and perhaps revising your technique.

The *Shiatzu* Routine

Remember: When working on an acupoint, first warm up the area with light rubbing, then apply appropriately moderate to heavy pressure, finishing with a soothing light rub.

Start with your partner lying face up. Proceed in the order described below.

Abdomen and Chest

Finger circles *(AN)*, finger stroking *(TUI)* and thumb pressure *(MO)* on:

Vc.6: along the front midline, two fingers below the navel (Vc.8)

Vc.12: pit of stomach halfway from the bottom of the breastbone (Vc.16) to the navel (Vc.8)

Vc.17: on the breastbone midline at the level of the nipples

Lg.1: on the chest one thumb below the collarbone midpoint, separate the muscle, between ribs

Neck

Finger stroking (move the skin over muscles), finger circles and finger pressure on:

Gb.21: uppermost part of the shoulder along the ridge, a finger from the neck toward the arm

Bl.10: near nape of the neck (Gv.15) two fingers to the side of midline

Gb.20: base of the skull about three fingers to the side of the midline (Gv.15)

Gv.15: base of skull on midline in hollow between the uppermost neck vertebra and the skull

Gv.16: about a finger width above the nape of the neck (Gv.15) in a notch below a bump

Head

Finger stroking on the scalp and finger pressure on:

Bl.2: on the face in a notch below the bushy part of the eyebrow

St.3: on the face one finger to the side of the nose at the level of the base of the nose

S-3: midway between the eyebrows under a bony ridge

S-9: on side of the face, a finger from the eye socket toward the ear, on a cord-like structure

Gv.20: on the scalp midline, halfway from the base of the skull (Gv.15) and the front hairline

Shoulder

Muscle pinching *(NA)*, finger stroking and thumb pressure on:

Gb.21: uppermost part of the shoulder along the ridge, a finger from the neck toward the arm

Have your partner turn face down. Continue shoulder movements to back of shoulders and upper back, finger circles, thumb stroking, muscle pinching and thumb pressure on:

Si.11: in the middle of the triangular shoulder blade

Arms

Muscle pinching, alternate pinching and thumb pressure on:

Co.10: between the forearm muscles, four fingers distance from the bony bump near the elbow

Cs.6: on the inside of the forearm 2.5 fingers from the wrist fold nearest the palm

Hand

Thumb circles and thumb pressure on:
Co.4: on the hand in the middle of the triangular web between the thumb and index finger

Back

(If you are right-handed, sit to the right of your partner.)
Finger circles (three times from neck down to sacrum, each side), heel of hand circles, thumb stroking and thumb pressure on:
Bl.11: upper back two fingers to side of back midline at the level of T1 vertebra
Bl.17: mid back two fingers to side of back midline, level with the lower tip of shoulder blade
Bl.26: low back two fingers to side of back midline, in a hollow above sacrum, below waistline

Hip

Alternate pinching, finger circles, heel of hand circles, thumb stroking and thumb pressure on:
Gb.30: in buttocks, from base of sacrum two-thirds distance toward the greater trochanter
S-74: in buttocks four fingers above Gb.30 and four fingers below the hipbone (iliac crest)

Back of Leg

Alternate pinching, finger circles, heel of hand circles, thumb stroking and thumb pressure on:

Bl.37: back of thigh halfway between the soft spot above the knee and the buttock fold

Bl.57: back of calf midline, halfway between the knee crease and tip of the external ankle

Have your partner turn face up to work on front side of legs.

Front of Legs

Muscle pinching, alternate pinching, thumb stroking and thumb pressure on:

Sp.6: inside the calf, four fingers above the tip of the anklebone

St.36: four fingers below the kneecap, in a muscle separation, one finger outside the shinbone

Sp.10: two fingers above the kneecap, inside the thigh near the edge of a muscle

Complete the circuit by rubbing the abdomen. See if the abdomen is less tender. Massage the neck using finger stroking and finger circles.

Acupressure Therapy

Since acupressure is an art, these therapeutic suggestions that I list are not definitive prescriptions for the various ailments listed below. How to press the acupoints or which formula to use is a matter of style. The goal is to benefit your partner with the least amount of discomfort.

When your partner presents a particular ailment, give a treatment that emphasizes the acupoints listed for that ailment. You might begin with those acupoints, come back to them in the middle of the *Shiatzu* routine and finish the treatment with the therapeutic acupoints once more.

A recipe for healing is choose the ingredients (points and strokes) then stir.

Anemia
(iron deficiency)

Improve diet, add whole grains and dark green vegetables if absent.

To improve absorption of iron, press:

St.36: four fingers below the kneecap, in a muscle separation, one finger outside the shinbone

Bl.17: mid back two fingers to side of back midline, level with the lower tip of shoulder blade

To strengthen the effect, select and press one or more:

Co.10: between the forearm muscles, four fingers distance from the bony bump near the elbow

Bl.11: upper back two fingers to side of back midline at the level of T1 vertebra

Bl.20: mid back two fingers to side of back midline at the level of T11 vertebra

Bl.23: low back two fingers to side of back midline at the level of L2 vertebra

Asthma
(difficulty breathing and wheezing)
See Lung Capacity

To stop attack, press:

Vc.17: on the breastbone midline at the level of the nipples
Vc.22: above the breastbone between the collarbones
Bl.11: upper back two fingers to side of back midline at the level of T1 vertebra

For infection, press:

Co.4: on the hand in the middle of the triangular web between the thumb and index finger
Co.10: between the forearm muscles, four fingers distance from the bony bump near the elbow

Between attacks, rub back and neck, then press:

Lg.1: on the chest one thumb below the collarbone midpoint, separate the muscle, between ribs
Vc.6: along the front midline, two fingers below the navel (Vc.8)
St.36: four fingers below the kneecap, in a muscle separation, one finger outside the shinbone
Bl.13: upper back two fingers to side of back midline at the level of T3 vertebra

Back Pain
See Sciatica

Pain means caution: energy at work.

First press *Ahshi* acupoints (tender spots) then press:

Bl.11: upper back two fingers to side of back midline at the level of T1 vertebra
Bl.17: mid back two fingers to side of back midline, level with the lower tip of shoulder blade

Bl.26: low back two fingers to side of back midline, in a hollow above sacrum, below waistline

Bl.37: back of thigh halfway between the soft spot above the knee and the buttock fold

Bl.57: back of calf midline, halfway between the knee crease and tip of the external ankle

To increase the effect, select and press one or more:

Vc.6: along the front midline, two fingers below the navel (Vc.8)

Bl.27: on the sacrum one fingers below Bl.26

Bl.28: on the sacrum two fingers below Bl.26

Gb.30: in buttocks, from base of sacrum two-thirds distance toward the greater trochanter

S-74: in buttocks four fingers above Gb.30 and four fingers below the hipbone (iliac crest)

Bed-wetting

For children more than five years old and some adults.
Rub the abdomen and press:

Vc.6: along the front midline, two fingers below the navel (Vc.8)

Sp.6: inside the calf, four fingers above the tip of the anklebone

For urinary bladder weakness, rub legs and back, press:

Bl.23: low back two fingers to side of back midline at the level of L2 vertebra

Bl.26: low back two fingers to side of back midline, in a hollow above sacrum, below waistline

Bl.28: on the sacrum two fingers below Bl.26

Bladder Infection

Eliminate *Yin* sweet foods, drink cranberry juice and/or potato water (water in which potatoes have been simmered).
To relieve irritation, press:

Vc.6: along the front midline, two fingers below the navel (Vc.8)

Bl.26: low back two fingers to side of back midline, in a hollow above sacrum, below waistline

Sp.6: inside the calf, four fingers above the tip of the anklebone

To strengthen bladder, press:

Bl.23: low back two fingers to side of back midline at the level of L2 vertebra

Bl.28: on the sacrum two fingers below Bl.26

Childbirth
See Pregnancy and Milk Flow

Trust and nurture your body. Listen to your body; it reflects nature. Love it; it was entrusted to you for its care and feeding. Nurture trust and trust nature.

Avoid cold food (raw food and fruit).

Give general back treatment and press:

St.36: four fingers below the kneecap, in a muscle separation, one finger outside the shinbone

Bl.26: low back two fingers to side of back midline, in a hollow above sacrum, below waistline

Gb.21: uppermost part of the shoulder along the ridge, a finger from the neck toward the arm

For difficult labor, press:

Co.4: on the hand in the middle of the triangular web between the thumb and index finger

Sp.6: inside the calf, four fingers above the tip of the anklebone

Bl.26: low back two fingers to side of back midline, in a hollow above sacrum, below waistline

To strengthen the effect of the above points, select and press one or more:

St.36: four fingers below the kneecap, in a muscle separation, one finger outside the shinbone

Bl.27: on the sacrum one finger below Bl.26

Bl.28: on the sacrum two fingers below Bl.26

Constipation

(Bowel movements should be once a day, in the morning.)

Improve diet. About ninety percent of your diet should be whole grains and vegetables.

Rub the abdomen especially in the morning before bowel movement. Press:

Vc.6: along the front midline, two fingers below the navel (Vc.8)

St.25: three fingers to the side of the navel

Vc.12: pit of stomach halfway from the bottom of the breastbone (Vc.16) to the navel (Vc.8)

Bl.57: back of calf midline, halfway between the knee crease and tip of the external ankle

Press on alternate days:

Yang days

Bl.26: low back two fingers to side of back midline, in a hollow above sacrum, below waistline

S-74: in buttocks four fingers above Gb.30 and four fingers below the hipbone (iliac crest)

Yin days

St.36: four fingers below the kneecap, in a muscle separation, one finger outside the shinbone

Co.4: on the hand in the middle of the triangular web between the thumb and index finger

Cough
See Sinusitis and Sore Throat

Rub back and neck. Press:

Lg.1: on the chest one thumb below the collarbone midpoint, separate the muscle, between ribs

St.36: four fingers below the kneecap, in a muscle separation, one finger outside the shinbone

Co.4: on the hand in the middle of the triangular web between the thumb and index finger

For congestion, press:

Bl.11: upper back two fingers to side of back midline at the level of T1 vertebra

Bl.17: mid back two fingers to side of back midline, level with the lower tip of shoulder blade

Co.10: between the forearm muscles, four fingers distance from the bony bump near the elbow

For dry, sore throat, press:

Vc.17: on the breastbone midline at the level of the nipples

Bl.11: upper back two fingers to side of back midline at the level of T1 vertebra

Vc.22: above the breastbone, between the collarbones

For nervous cough, press:

Vc.22: above the breastbone, between the collarbones

Depression

See Mental Disorder

(when not complicated by mental disorder)

Rub back and press:

Vc.6: along the front midline, two fingers below the navel (Vc.8)

Cs.6: on the inside of the forearm 2.5 fingers from the wrist fold nearest the palm

Bl.10: near nape of the neck (Gv.15) two fingers to the side of midline

Gv.20: on the scalp midline, halfway from the base of the skull (Gv.15) and the front hairline

Gv.16: about a finger width above the nape of the neck (Gv.15) in a notch below a bump

Gb.20: base of the skull about three fingers to the side of the midline (Gv.15)

St.36: four fingers below the kneecap, in a muscle separation, one finger outside the shinbone

Lg.1: on the chest one thumb below the collarbone midpoint, separate the muscle, between ribs

Diarrhea
See Stomachache and Digestion, Poor

Press:

Vc.12: pit of stomach halfway from the bottom of the breastbone (Vc.16) to the navel (Vc.8)

Co.10: between the forearm muscles, four fingers distance from the bony bump near the elbow

Co.4: on the hand in the middle of the triangular web between the thumb and index finger

St.36: four fingers below the kneecap, in a muscle separation, one finger outside the shinbone

For chronic diarrhea, press:

Bl.20: mid back two fingers to side of back midline at the level of T11 vertebra

Sp.6: inside the calf, four fingers above the tip of the anklebone

Digestion, Poor
See Stomachache, Constipation and Diarrhea

It may be necessary to change the diet. The following will help.

Rub the abdomen and press:

St.36: four fingers below the kneecap, in a muscle separation, one finger outside the shinbone

Sp.6: inside the calf, four fingers above the tip of the anklebone

Bl.26: low back two fingers to side of back midline, in a hollow above sacrum, below waistline

Vc.12: pit of stomach halfway from the bottom of the breastbone (Vc.16) to the navel (Vc.8)

To strengthen the effect, press one or more:

Co.4: on the hand in the middle of the triangular web between the thumb and index finger

Co.10: between the forearm muscles, four fingers distance from the bony bump near the elbow

Cs.6: on the inside of the forearm 2.5 fingers from the wrist fold nearest the palm

Bl.20: mid back two fingers to side of back midline at the level of T11 vertebra

Bl.23: low back two fingers to side of back midline at the level of L2 vertebra

Dizziness
See Shock and Fainting

Press:

Gv.16: about a finger width above the nape of the neck (Gv.15) in a notch below a bump

Gb.20: base of the skull about three fingers to the side of the midline (Gv.15)

S-9: on side of the face, a finger from the eye socket toward the ear, on a cord-like structure

Eye Problems

(caused by excess alcohol, sun, wind, or strain)

Wash with a cool one percent salt water solution to soothe the eyes.

For eyestrain, press:

Bl.2: on the face in a notch below the bushy part of the eyebrow

Gb.20: base of the skull about three fingers to the side of the midline (Gv.15)

Bl.10: near nape of the neck (Gv.15) two fingers to the side of midline

For red swollen eyes, press:

Co.4: on the hand in the middle of the triangular web between the thumb and index finger

S-9: on side of the face, a finger from the eye socket toward the ear, on a cord-like structure

Facial Beauty

A good complexion is a sign of health. Avoid excess sun.

Relax face, press:

S-3: midway between the eyebrows under a bony ridge

Bl.2: on the face in a notch below the bushy part of the eyebrow

S-9: on side of the face, a finger from the eye socket toward the ear, on a cord-like structure

St.3: on the face one finger to the side of the nose at the level of the base of the nose

To improve skin, press:

Lg.1: on the chest one thumb below the collarbone midpoint, separate the muscle, between ribs

Co.4: on the hand in the middle of the triangular web between the thumb and index finger

St.36: four fingers below the kneecap, in a muscle separation, one finger outside the shinbone

Fatigue

Always a serious sign of lost health.

Rub feet, press:

Vc.6: along the front midline, two fingers below the navel (Vc.8)

Co.4: on the hand in the middle of the triangular web between the thumb and index finger

St.36: four fingers below the kneecap, in a muscle separation, one finger outside the shinbone

For physical fatigue, press:

Vc.12: pit of stomach halfway from the bottom of the breastbone (Vc.16) to the navel (Vc.8)

Cs.6: on the inside of the forearm 2.5 fingers from the wrist fold nearest the palm

Co.10: between the forearm muscles, four fingers distance from the bony bump near the elbow

For mental fatigue, press:

Gb.20: base of the skull about three fingers to the side of the midline (Gv.15)

Gv.16: about a finger width above the nape of the neck (Gv.15) in a notch below a bump

Gv.20: on the scalp midline, halfway from the base of the skull (Gv.15) and the front hairline

Fever

Combine with treatment for other symptoms as appropriate.

Press:

Co.4: on the hand in the middle of the triangular web between the thumb and index finger

Sp.10: two fingers above the kneecap, inside the thigh near the edge of a muscle

Co.10: between the forearm muscles, four fingers distance from the bony bump near the elbow

Headache
See Migraine, Neckache and Toothache

Pain is not a predicament—it is a process.

Look for deeper problems.

Rub neck, head and shoulders, then press:

Co.4: on the hand in the middle of the triangular web between the thumb and index finger

214

Bl.2: on the face in a notch below the bushy part of the eyebrow

Press on alternate days:

Yang days

S-9: on side of the face, a finger from the eye socket toward the ear, on a cord-like structure

Gv.20: on the scalp midline, halfway from the base of the skull (Gv.15) and the front hairline

Bl.10: near nape of the neck (Gv.15) two fingers to the side of midline

Yin days

S-3: midway between the eyebrows under a bony ridge

Gv.15: base of skull on midline in hollow between the uppermost neck vertebra and the skull

St.36: four fingers below the kneecap, in a muscle separation, one finger outside the shinbone

Hemorrhoids

Treat other symptoms. Look for a deeper cause.

Rub *Hara,* lower back and press:

Gv.20: on the scalp midline, halfway from the base of the skull (Gv.15) and the front hairline

Bl.57: back of calf midline, halfway between the knee crease and tip of the external ankle

Hiccoughs

Press:

Cs.6: on the inside of the forearm 2.5 fingers from the wrist fold nearest the palm

Bl.17: mid back two fingers to side of back midline, level with the lower tip of shoulder blade

Vc.22: above the breastbone, between the collarbones

Hypertension
(high blood pressure)

Acupressure is excellent for primary hypertension, which is a stress-induced disorder, which can lead to many problems if not corrected. Avoid excess emotion. Balance a physical exercise program with periods of relaxation. Avoid alcohol, caffeine and stimulants.

Press:

S-3: midway between the eyebrows under a bony ridge

St.36: four fingers below the kneecap, in a muscle separation, one finger outside the shinbone

Co.10: between the forearm muscles, four fingers distance from the bony bump near the elbow

Bl.57: back of calf midline, halfway between the knee crease and tip of the external ankle

Secondary hypertension stems from many causes. See a physician if necessary.

Press:

Co.10: between the forearm muscles, four fingers distance from the bony bump near the elbow

St.36: four fingers below the kneecap, in a muscle separation, one finger outside the shinbone

Press on alternate days:

Yang days

Gb.21: uppermost part of the shoulder along the ridge, a finger from the neck toward the arm

Gb.20: base of the skull about three fingers to the side of the midline (Gv.15)

Yin days

Bl.10: near nape of the neck (Gv.15) two fingers to the side of midline

Vc.17: on the breastbone midline at the level of the nipples

Injuries

Pain is not a predicament—it is a process.

Use local acupoints and distant acupoints on the opposite side of the body from the injury.

Press:

St.36: four fingers below the kneecap, in a muscle separation, one finger outside the shinbone

Vc.6: along the front midline, two fingers below the navel (Vc.8)

For burns, bruises, add:

Lg.1: on the chest one thumb below the collarbone midpoint, separate the muscle, between ribs

Sp.10: two fingers above the kneecap, inside the thigh near the edge of a muscle

For strain, sprain, add:

Sp.6: inside the calf, four fingers above the tip of the anklebone

Bl.57: back of calf midline, halfway between the knee crease and tip of the external ankle

For bone injuries, press:

Bl.11: upper back two fingers to side of back midline at the level of T1 vertebra

For pain, press:

Co.4: on the hand in the middle of the triangular web between the thumb and index finger

St.36: four fingers below the kneecap, in a muscle separation, one finger outside the shinbone

Insomnia

Press in series:

S-3: midway between the eyebrows under a bony ridge

Bl.10: near nape of the neck (Gv.15) two fingers to the side of midline

Lg.1: on the chest one thumb below the collarbone midpoint, separate the muscle, between ribs

Bl.2: on the face in a notch below the bushy part of the eyebrow

Cs.6: on the inside of the forearm 2.5 fingers from the wrist fold nearest the palm

Sp.6: inside the calf, four fingers above the tip of the anklebone

Due to active mind, press:

Vc.6: along the front midline, two fingers below the navel (Vc.8)

Gv.20: on the scalp midline, halfway from the base of the skull (Gv.15) and the front hairline

Longevity

An ancient saying is "To live a long life, sweat every day."
Rub every day:

Co.4: on the hand in the middle of the triangular web between the thumb and index finger

St.36: four fingers below the kneecap, in a muscle separation, one finger outside the shinbone

Vc.6: along the front midline, two fingers below the navel (Vc.8)

Bl.26: low back two fingers to side of back midline, in a hollow above sacrum, below waistline

Lung Capacity

To increase breath capacity, press:

Bl.11: upper back two fingers to side of back midline at the level of T1 vertebra

Bl.17: mid back two fingers to side of back midline, level with the lower tip of shoulder blade

Co.4: on the hand in the middle of the triangular web between the thumb and index finger

Memory

Press:

Gv.20: on the scalp midline, halfway from the base of the skull (Gv.15) and the front hairline

218

Vc.12: pit of stomach halfway from the bottom of the breastbone (Vc.16) to the navel (Vc.8)

Cs.6: on the inside of the forearm 2.5 fingers from the wrist fold nearest the palm

Menstrual Problems
See Vaginal Problems

Rub *Hara*, back, inside legs, press:

Vc.6: along the front midline, two fingers below the navel (Vc.8)

Sp.6: inside the calf, four fingers above the tip of the anklebone

For pain press firmly until gone:

Co.4: on the hand in the middle of the triangular web between the thumb and index finger

Sp.6: inside the calf, four fingers above the tip of the anklebone

Sp.10: two fingers above the kneecap, inside the thigh near the edge of a muscle

For swelling, add:

Sp.6: inside the calf, four fingers above the tip of the anklebone

Lg.1: on the chest one thumb below the collarbone midpoint, separate the muscle, between ribs

Bl.26: low back two fingers to side of back midline, in a hollow above sacrum, below waistline

For depression, press:

Vc.6: along the front midline, two fingers below the navel (Vc.8)

Vc.12: pit of stomach halfway from the bottom of the breastbone (Vc.16) to the navel (Vc.8)

Sp.6: inside the calf, four fingers above the tip of the anklebone

For cramps, press:

Sp.6: inside the calf, four fingers above the tip of the anklebone

Bl.57: back of calf midline, halfway between the knee crease and tip of the external ankle

Irregular, add:

(evening)

Bl.26: low back two fingers to side of back midline, in a hollow above sacrum, below waistline

Vc.12: pit of stomach halfway from the bottom of the breastbone (Vc.16) to the navel (Vc.8)

Sp.6: inside the calf, four fingers above the tip of the anklebone
   (morning)

St.36: four fingers below the kneecap, in a muscle separation, one finger outside the shinbone

Vc.6: along the front midline, two fingers below the navel (Vc.8)

Sp.10: two fingers above the kneecap, inside the thigh near the edge of a muscle
   (during the day)

Sp.6: inside the calf, four fingers above the tip of the anklebone

Bl.57: back of calf midline, halfway between the knee crease and tip of the external ankle

Mental Disorder
See Depression when not associated with a mental disorder

Physical exercise and wholesome diet are recommended.

Rub neck and back, press:

Vc.12: pit of stomach halfway from the bottom of the breastbone (Vc.16) to the navel (Vc.8)

Vc.17: on the breastbone midline at the level of the nipples

Gv.20: on the scalp midline, halfway from the base of the skull (Gv.15) and the front hairline

Migraine
See Headache

Commonly triggered by allergies
During attack, press firmly:

Co.4: on the hand in the middle of the triangular web between the thumb and index finger

Co.10: between the forearm muscles, four fingers distance from the bony bump near the elbow

Vc.6: along the front midline, two fingers below the navel (Vc.8)

Lv.3: on top of the foot between the longest bones on the foot

Select, according to area affected:

Front:

Bl.2: on the face in a notch below the bushy part of the eyebrow

S-9: on side of the face, a finger from the eye socket toward the ear, on a cord-like structure

St.36: four fingers below the kneecap, in a muscle separation, one finger outside the shinbone

Side:

Gb.20: base of the skull about three fingers to the side of the midline (Gv.15)

S-9: on side of the face, a finger from the eye socket toward the ear, on a cord-like structure

Gb.21: uppermost part of the shoulder along the ridge, a finger from the neck toward the arm

Back:

Bl.10: near nape of the neck (Gv.15) two fingers to the side of midline

Gv.15: base of skull on midline in hollow between the uppermost neck vertebra and the skull

Bl.26: low back two fingers to side of back midline, in a hollow above sacrum, below waistline

Gv.20: on the scalp midline, halfway from the base of the skull (Gv.15) and the front hairline

Between attacks, rub neck and back, press:

Vc.6: along the front midline, two fingers below the navel (Vc.8)

St.36: four fingers below the kneecap, in a muscle separation, one finger outside the shinbone

Co.4: on the hand in the middle of the triangular web between the thumb and index finger

Vc.17: on the breastbone midline at the level of the nipples

Milk Flow

No milk flow, press:

Vc.17: on the breastbone midline at the level of the nipples

Gb.21: uppermost part of the shoulder along the ridge, a finger from the neck toward the arm

To strengthen the effect of the above points, select and press one or more:

Bl.17: mid back two fingers to side of back midline, level with the lower tip of shoulder blade

Bl.18: mid back two fingers to side of back midline, level with the T9 vertebra

Bl.20: mid back two fingers to side of back midline, level with the T11 vertebra

St.36: four fingers below the kneecap, in a muscle separation, one finger outside the shinbone

Nausea
See Pregnancy

To induce vomiting, press deep:

Vc.22: above the breastbone, between the collarbones

To prevent, press:

Cs.6: on the inside of the forearm 2.5 fingers from the wrist fold nearest the palm

Vc.17: on the breastbone midline at the level of the nipples

St.36: four fingers below the kneecap, in a muscle separation, one finger outside the shinbone

Follow up by pressing for three days:

Vc.17: on the breastbone midline at the level of the nipples

Vc.12: pit of stomach halfway from the bottom of the breastbone (Vc.16) to the navel (Vc.8)

Vc.6: along the front midline, two fingers below the navel (Vc.8)

Neckache
See Headache and Backache

Pain means caution: energy at work.

Repeat sequence of acupoints seated or lying, whichever is the most comfortable.

While seated, rub neck and shoulders, press:

Gb.20: base of the skull about three fingers to the side of the midline (Gv.15)

Bl.10: near nape of the neck (Gv.15) two fingers to the side of midline

Bl.11: upper back two fingers to side of back midline at the level of T1 vertebra

Gb.21: uppermost part of the shoulder along the ridge, a finger from the neck toward the arm

While lying on belly, rub back and press:

Bl.11: upper back two fingers to side of back midline at the level of T1 vertebra

Bl.17: mid back two fingers to side of back midline, level with the lower tip of shoulder blade

Bl.26: low back two fingers to side of back midline, in a hollow above sacrum, below waistline

Si.11: in the middle of the triangular shoulder blade

Nosebleed

To stop immediately, pull the hairs at the nape of the neck near acupoints Bl.10 and Gv.15. If this fails to stop the bleeding, press and hold the side of the nose gently.

To prevent chronic nosebleed, press daily for ten days:

Bl.10: near nape of the neck (Gv.15) two fingers to the side of midline

Co.4: on the hand in the middle of the triangular web between the thumb and index finger

St.36: four fingers below the kneecap, in a muscle separation, one finger outside the shinbone

Numbness
See Stroke and Sciatica

Treat as soon as possible to prevent permanent nerve damage.

Press local and other sensitive acupoints.

Select from the following:

Gv.16: about a finger width above the nape of the neck (Gv.15) in a notch below a bump

Si.11: in the middle of the triangular shoulder blade

Cs.6: on the inside of the forearm 2.5 fingers from the wrist fold nearest the palm

S-74: in buttocks four fingers above Gb.30 and four fingers below the hipbone (iliac crest)

Bl.17: mid back two fingers to side of back midline, level with the lower tip of shoulder blade

Pain and Stiffness
See other symptoms as appropriate

Pain means caution: energy at work.

Pain is the body's way of saying something is wrong. Look for the source. If it is *internal,* other means beside acupressure may be necessary to correct the disorder. Press *Ahshi* acupoints (tender spots) and acupoints along the *meridians* that go through the painful area.

Also select from the following:

Co.4: on the hand in the middle of the triangular web between the thumb and index finger

St.36: four fingers below the kneecap, in a muscle separation, one finger outside the shinbone

224

For abdominal pain, add:

Sp.6: inside the calf, four fingers above the tip of the anklebone

For arthritis, add:

Co.10: between the forearm muscles, four fingers distance from the bony bump near the elbow

Gb.30: in buttocks, from base of sacrum two-thirds distance toward the greater trochanter

For rheumatism, add:

St.3: on the face one finger to the side of the nose at the level of the base of the nose

Pregnancy
See Childbirth and Milk Flow

Avoid cold food (raw food and fruit). During pregnancy, exercise back and legs.

Give general back treatment and press:

St.36: four fingers below the kneecap, in a muscle separation, one finger outside the shinbone

Bl.26: low back two fingers to side of back midline, in a hollow above sacrum, below waistline

Gb.21: uppermost part of the shoulder along the ridge, a finger from the neck toward the arm

For nausea, press:

Cs.6: on the inside of the forearm 2.5 fingers from the wrist fold nearest the palm

Vc.12: pit of stomach halfway from the bottom of the breastbone (Vc.16) to the navel (Vc.8)

Rash

A rash could indicate many other disorders.

Press local acupoints outside the affected area toward the trunk. Press:

Co.4: on the hand in the middle of the triangular web between the thumb and index finger
Sp.10: two fingers above the kneecap, inside the thigh near the edge of a muscle

Resistance to Disease

Keep your immune system strong.
Press:
Co.4: on the hand in the middle of the triangular web between the thumb and index finger
Co.10: between the forearm muscles, four fingers distance from the bony bump near the elbow
St.36: four fingers below the kneecap, in a muscle separation, one finger outside the shinbone

Sciatica

See Back Pain

When lower back pain radiates down the leg.
First press *Ahshi* acupoints (tender spots) then press:
Bl.26: low back two fingers to side of back midline, in a hollow above sacrum, below waistline
Gb.30: in buttocks, from base of sacrum two-thirds distance toward the greater trochanter
S-74: in buttocks four fingers above Gb.30 and four fingers below the hipbone (iliac crest)
Bl.37: back of thigh halfway between the soft spot above the knee and the buttock fold
Bl.57: back of calf midline, halfway between the knee crease and tip of the external ankle
To increase the effect, select and press one or more:
Bl.23: low back two fingers to side of back midline at the level of L2 vertebra
Vc.6: along the front midline, two fingers below the navel (Vc.8)

Bl.37: back of thigh halfway between the soft spot above the knee and the buttock fold

Bl.27: on the sacrum one fingers below Bl.26

Bl.28: on the sacrum two fingers below Bl.26

Sexual Vitality

Having sexual energy is a sign of health; learning to control it is a sign of maturity.

To generate, daily press:

Co.4: on the hand in the middle of the triangular web between the thumb and index finger

Sp.6: inside the calf, four fingers above the tip of the anklebone

To unblock, press:

Bl.26: low back two fingers to side of back midline, in a hollow above sacrum, below waistline

Gb.30: in buttocks, from base of sacrum two-thirds distance toward the greater trochanter

Vc.6: along the front midline, two fingers below the navel (Vc.8)

Add as necessary:

St.36: four fingers below the kneecap, in a muscle separation, one finger outside the shinbone

Bl.23: low back two fingers to side of back midline at the level of L2 vertebra

Try pressing on your partner during sex:

S-74: in buttocks four fingers above Gb.30 and four fingers below the hipbone (iliac crest)

Shock and Fainting
See Dizziness

Alternate rubbing and pressing until improved or appropriate medical treatment can be administered. Keep warm, loosen clothing and raise feet.

First press:

Gv.26: pinch the upper lip just under the nose

Cs.6: on the inside of the forearm 2.5 fingers from the wrist fold nearest the palm

    Rub:

Gv.20: on the scalp midline, halfway from the base of the skull (Gv.15) and the front hairline

Vc.6: along the front midline, two fingers below the navel (Vc.8)

Vc.12: pit of stomach halfway from the bottom of the breastbone (Vc.16) to the navel (Vc.8)

    Press:

St.36: four fingers below the kneecap, in a muscle separation, one finger outside the shinbone

Gv.26: pinch the upper lip just under the nose

Cs.6: on the inside of the forearm 2.5 fingers from the wrist fold nearest the palm

    To raise blood pressure, press hard:

Gv.25: pinch tip of nose

Ki.1: bottom of foot under Lv.3

Sinusitis
See Cough and Sore Throat

    Press:

Co.10: between the forearm muscles, four fingers distance from the bony bump near the elbow

St.36: four fingers below the kneecap, in a muscle separation, one finger outside the shinbone

Gb.30: in buttocks, from base of sacrum two-thirds distance toward the greater trochanter

Gv.15: base of skull on midline in hollow between the uppermost neck vertebra and the skull

    For upper sinus, add:

Bl.2: on the face in a notch below the bushy part of the eyebrow

S-9: on side of the face, a finger from the eye socket toward the ear, on a cord-like structure

228

Bl.10: near nape of the neck (Gv.15) two fingers to the side of midline

For lower sinus, add:

St.3: on the face one finger to the side of the nose at the level of the base of the nose

Gb.20: base of the skull about three fingers to the side of the midline (Gv.15)

St.36: four fingers below the kneecap, in a muscle separation, one finger outside the shinbone

For nose add:

Co.4: on the hand in the middle of the triangular web between the thumb and index finger

S-3: midway between the eyebrows under a bony ridge

Bl.10: near nape of the neck (Gv.15) two fingers to the side of midline

Sore Throat
See Sinusitis and Cough

Pain is not a predicament—it is a process.

Press:

Co.4: on the hand in the middle of the triangular web between the thumb and index finger

Lg.1: on the chest one thumb below the collarbone midpoint, separate the muscle, between ribs

Bl.11: upper back two fingers to side of back midline at the level of T1 vertebra

For inflammation (tonsillitis), press:

Gv.15: base of skull on midline in hollow between the uppermost neck vertebra and the skull

Vc.22: above the breastbone, between the collarbones

For mucus, press:

Vc.17: on the breastbone midline at the level of the nipples

Gb.20: base of the skull about three fingers to the side of the midline (Gv.15)

For dry throat, press:

St.36: four fingers below the kneecap, in a muscle separation, one finger outside the shinbone

Sp.6: inside the calf, four fingers above the tip of the anklebone

Stomachache
See Constipation and Diarrhea

Improve the diet and eat regularly.

Rub the abdomen and shoulders. Press:

Vc.12: pit of stomach halfway from the bottom of the breastbone (Vc.16) to the navel (Vc.8)

Cs.6: on the inside of the forearm 2.5 fingers from the wrist fold nearest the palm

St.36: four fingers below the kneecap, in a muscle separation, one finger outside the shinbone

Co.10: between the forearm muscles, four fingers distance from the bony bump near the elbow

For cramps, press three times daily:

Si.11: in the middle of the triangular shoulder blade

Bl.57: back of calf midline, halfway between the knee crease and tip of the external ankle

For spasm, press:

Bl.17: mid back two fingers to side of back midline, level with the lower tip of shoulder blade

Bl.26: low back two fingers to side of back midline, in a hollow above sacrum, below waistline

Stroke
See Numbness

Apply acupressure with other forms of therapy.

Give general acupressure massage; emphasize local points. Press:

Gv.16: about a finger width above the nape of the neck (Gv.15) in a notch below a bump

Gv.20: on the scalp midline, halfway from the base of the skull (Gv.15) and the front hairline

Toothache
See Headache

A change in diet may be indicated.

Until the appropriate treatment is obtained, press:

Co.4: on the hand in the middle of the triangular web between the thumb and index finger

Co.10: between the forearm muscles, four fingers distance from the bony bump near the elbow

St.3: on the face one finger to the side of the nose at the level of the base of the nose

Vaginal Problems
See Menstrual Problems

Eliminate meat and sugar until relieved.

For itch, press:

Sp.6: inside the calf, four fingers above the tip of the anklebone

Sp.10: two fingers above the kneecap, inside the thigh near the edge of a muscle

For pain, press:

Vc.6: along the front midline, two fingers below the navel (Vc.8)

Sp.6: inside the calf, four fingers above the tip of the anklebone

Co.4: on the hand in the middle of the triangular web between the thumb and index finger

For swelling, press:

Sp.10: two fingers above the kneecap, inside the thigh near the edge of a muscle

For discharge, press:

Vc.6: along the front midline, two fingers below the navel (Vc.8)

Sp.6: inside the calf, four fingers above the tip of the anklebone

St.36: four fingers below the kneecap, in a muscle separation, one finger outside the shinbone

Sp.10: two fingers above the kneecap, inside the thigh near the edge of a muscle

Appendix

Fuxi's Biography by Confucius

After visiting many imperial libraries, Confucius (b. -551, d. -479) popularized several books including the *I Ching (Classic of Change)*. He studied the book for its wisdom and discouraged using it for divination. The *I Ching* evolved from the practice of oracle bone divination (the most ancient evidence for Chinese writing and the theory of yinyang). The mythical Fuxi (伏羲 sounds like "foo sheh," means animal tamer) is mentioned by Confucius in his *Grand Commentary* to the *I Ching, (Yijing Tachuan)*. Ancient texts are often difficult to read because of the terse nature of ancient Chinese writing. The following literal translation has clarifying comments in parentheses.

> The ancients indicated the Xi clan (Fuxi) had a king (ruled the world) below heaven, looking up, he saw patterns and images in Heaven (stars, weather), looking down, he saw patterns and methods on Earth (laws of nature), he saw birds and beasts had word helps on Earth have suitability, (Observing the birds and beasts communicating on Earth, he understood the meaning) his body could grasp (sense) all that is near and, all things left records (signs) so he could grasp (sense) at a distance, the Eight Trigrams are a good place to start, use it to reach illuminating insights, it has virtue, use it to group innumerable things, it has categories. He made knotted cords (used in record keeping) and snare nets, for use in the field (to capture and tame animals) and in fishing.

Want to try your hand at translating Chinese? Nowadays, Chinese text is written from left to right and from top to bottom. Look for word patterns. Organizing words (er2, ye3, yi3, yu2, zhe3, zhi1) are often used to indicate word patterns. Phrases (ze2 guan1, qu3 zhu1) are also used to form patterns in this text. The following text is organized to make the word patterns easier to see. Try different meanings of a word. Add different English organizing words (the, in, on, that, for, etc.). Try different word combinations. You may come up with a new way to translate this text. Actually it is common for ancient philosophical texts to have multiple meanings.

Fuxi's biography by Confucius

古者戲氏之王天下也，
gu3 zhe3 xi4 shi4 zhi1 wang2 tian1 xia4 ye3,

仰則觀象於天，
yang3 ze2 guan1 xiang4 zhi1 tian1 yu2,

俯則觀法於地，
fu3 ze2 guan1 fa3 yu2 di4,

觀鳥獸之文與地之宜，
guan1 niao3 shou4 zhi1 wen2 yu3 di4 zhi1 yi2,

近取諸身，遠取諸物，
jin4 qu3 zhu1 shen1, yuan3 qu3 zhu1 wu4,

於是始作八卦，
yu2 shi4 shi3 zuo4 ba1 gua4,

以達神明之德，
yi3 da2 shen2 ming2 zhi1 de2,

以類萬物之情。
yi3 lei4 wan4 wu4 zhi1 qing2.

作結繩而為 … 以田以漁。
zuo4 jie2 sheng2 er2 wei2 … yi3 tian2 yi3 yu2.

Abbreviated Dictionary
For use with Fuxi Text

八 ba1 — eight

達 da2 reach — extend; reach; understandable; express; distinguished

德 de2 virtue — virtue, moral, ethics; kindness

地 di4 earth — Earth; land, ground, field; place

而 er2 and — (conjunction) and, but, yet, etc.

法 fa3 method — law; method; model after

俯 fu3 bow — bow, condescend

古 gu3 ancient — ancient, age-old

罟 gu3 snare net — a net; a drag-net; involved, implicate

卦 gua4 trigrams — divination symbol

觀 guan1 view — look at, to view; a view; outlook, point of view

結 jie2 knotted — knot, knit, weave; consolidate, form; settle

近 jin4 near — near, close; approaching; intimate

類 lei4 group — type, category; resemble; similar to

明 ming2 clear — bright; clear; open, explicit; know, understand

鳥 niao3 bird

情 qing2 feeling — feeling; love; passion; favor; situation; kind

取 qu3 grasp — grasp, take, get; receive; choose, seek, select

身 shen1 body — body, person; trunk; life

神 shen2 insight — God, divine; spirit, mind; expression, look; smart

繩 sheng2 cord — cord, rope, string; restrain

始 shi3 start, first — beginning, start; only then

氏 shi4 — clan; Mr. Mrs.

是 shi4 true — correct; yes; this, that; is, was, to be

獸 shou4 beasts — beast, animal; brutal

天 tian1 heaven — sky, heaven; day; weather; season; God

田 tian2 farm — field, farmland

萬 wan4 myriad — ten thousand; myriad

王 wang2 ruler — king, ruler

爲 wei2 become — cause; become; to do; to be

文 wen2 writing — literature; Chinese characters; language; civil; sign of nature

物 wu4 things — thing, matter; macrocosm; substance; content

戲 xi4 — Fuxi's (伏羲) clan

下 xia4 below — below, down; next; under; inferior

象 xiang4 image — elephant; image; imitate; resemble

仰 yang3 lookup — look upward; respect, admire; rely on

也 ye3 also — also, too, either

宜 yi2 proper — suitable, appropriate; should

以 yi3 use — use; according to; because of; in order to

漁 yu2 fish — fish, fishing

於 yu2 in — (indicates comparison/connection) with, at, to, in, than

與 yu3 give — give; help; offer; and

遠 yuan3 far — far, remote, distant

則 ze2 model — standard, rule; pattern; imitate

者 zhe3 — (indicates a pronoun) this, here

之 zhi1 possesses — (indicates possession) his, hers; this, that; goes

諸 zhu1 all — all, various; put into practice

作 zuo4 — compose, make - do, make; rise; write, compose; affect, feel

The Yellow Sovereign on the Cause of Pain

The *Yellow Sovereign's Classic* is the oldest evidence for the Oriental understanding that pain is injured *Qi* energy. The following translation is stylized to teach the principle of yinyang, covered in the first twenty percent of chapter five.

The Yellow Sovereign's Classic of Internal Medicine
Huangdi Neijing, Suwen
黄帝内經素問

From Chapter 5
Grand Theory on the Reciprocal Nature of Yinyang
Yinyang Yingxiang Dalun
陰陽應像大論

The Yellow Sovereign said: *Yinyang* follows the way *(DAO* 道) of Heaven and Earth. It is the basic principle of change, the mother of all. It is a treasury of illuminating insights (神明 *SHENMING).* Making and breaking begins at the root. To cure disease you must seek and destroy the root.

Heaven (weather) typifies restless *yang,* which grows and weakens; Earth typifies quiet *yin,* which nurtures and stores. *Yang* transforms *Qi* (bio-energy); *yin* structures matter (the body). Cold extremes produce heat; heat extremes produce cold. Cold *Qi* produces muddiness (cold air is foggy and cold weather makes snow), hot *Qi* produces clarity (hot desert air is clear and hot air purifies metal—the refiner's fire). Similarly, cleansing *Qi* afflicts below (in the bowels) producing diarrhea; muddy *Qi* afflicts above (in the chest) producing congestion. Thus, *yinyang* fosters rebellion and a disease of opposition follows.

Heaven purifies like *yang;* Earth muddies like *yin.* Similarly Earth *Qi* rises (mist) to become clouds in heaven; *Qi* then falls as rain. Rain comes out of Earth *Qi*; clouds come out of Heaven *Qi*.

(The *yang-fire* of heaven purifies water by evaporation and condensation, which then rains, cooling the Earth, which then becomes muddy. The *yin-water* of Earth clouds (muddies) heaven by evaporation and condensation, which forms clouds, which obscure the sun or falls as rain water returning to earth.)

Similarly clear *yang* (breath) comes out of our upper orifices; muddy *yin* (urine and stool) comes out of our lower orifices. Clear (cleansing) *yang* responds through the pores (sweat, saliva and tears). Muddy *yin* goes to the five viscera (kidney, liver, heart, spleen, lung). Clear *yang* surplus (excess) fills the four limbs (arms and legs). Muddy *yin* goes into the six bowels (bladder, gall bladder, small intestine, large intestine, stomach, triple heater).

Water is *yin;* fire is *yang.*

Qi is *yang;* flavor (food) is *yin.*

Food (flavor) restores the body; the body restores *Qi* (energy); *Qi* restores *jing-essence; jing-essence* restores transformations (change); *Jing-essence* consumes *Qi,* the body consumes food (flavor); Transformation employs *jing-essence; Qi* generates (produces) the body.

Flavors (can) injure the body, *Qi* (can) injure the *jing-essence; Jing-essence* transformations are *Qi; Qi* is also injured by flavors. (Therefore, be careful: the food you eat can damage your body and deplete your energy. Change your lifestyle or you will limit your ability to change your life with style.)

Yin food (flavor) exits our lower orifices; *yang Qi* (breath) exits our upper orifices. Strong food (flavor) is *yin;* moderate (weak) (flavor) has *yang* for (balancing) *yin.* Strong *Qi* is *yang;* moderate (weak) *(Qi)* has *yin* for (balancing) *yang.*

Strong flavor (food) results in bowel movement disorders; mild is the way to go. Moderate (weak) *Qi* flows freely; strong *(Qi)* is too hot. Strong fire results in a weak *Qi;* less fire results in strong *Qi*. Strong fire consumes *Qi; Qi* consumes less (weak) fire. Strong fire scatters *Qi;* moderate (weak) fire produces *Qi.* Food *Qi,* when spicy hot and sweet (flavor), causes disorders and discharges of *yang* (fire); Sour and bitter (flavor) cause surges and purges of *yin* (water). *Yin* surplus results in *yang* diseases; *yang* surplus results in *yin* diseases. *Yang* surplus results in heat; *yin* surplus results in cold. Excessive cold results in heat; excessive heat results in cold. Cold injures the body; heat injures the *Qi; Qi* injuries hurt (pain is injured *Qi);* body injuries swell. Similarly, swelling after pain injures the body and pain after swelling injures the *Qi.*

Inductive and Deductive Logic

In the West we trust that which is rational; in the East they depend on that which is relational. We develop the intelligence; they develop the intuition. We study cause and effect; they study symbolic association.

The *yinyang* way of seeing is a scientific and logical way to examine things. It is, however, not the logical rational way taught in schools in the Western world, except for a few obscure courses in upper division logic. There are two systems of logic (duality again?): inductive and deductive. In deductive logic, the premise is followed by the conclusion, often referred to as cause and effect. We even say it is logical, but meaning deductively logical (as if inductive logic is illogical).

Inductive logic is another kind of logic that doesn't seem logical in modern Western thought. Inductive systems of logic are based on the notion that the part represents the whole. Or, stated another way, you can learn something of the whole by observing the parts. With inductive reasoning all the facts need not be accurate and you don't need to know all the information in order to draw a conclusion, but you cannot be certain that you are right. Close is often good enough. Inductive logic concerns itself with symbolic relationships rather than rational sequences. With deductive reasoning, if the facts and the premise are correct, then the conclusion can be relied upon.

As an example, consider a picture with a simple image of a shadow of a tree cast on a field. Inductively you could say it is day and the sun is shining. The shadow implies the existence of the tree behind the camera. The length of the shadow would indicate how close to morning, noon or evening it is. There is a source of water nearby. Depending on the type of tree we could imply whether the climate is warm or cold. Now none of this is certain. It could be a spot light and the tree could be a cardboard cutout. Deductively you could only make a qualified statement, "If I knew for sure that the camera is outdoors and no dummy trees are being used, then the tree blocks the light of the sun casting a shadow on the field."

Inductive logic seems to be the product of right brain **looking** rather than left brain **reasoning**. Which way is most logical? Is one right or wrong? It's interesting, but yinyang can't help us here. Of all the pairs the yin and yang are associated with, right and wrong are excluded. If there is a right or wrong to it, perhaps it is that we only use one kind of logic exclusively or perhaps it is wrong to think one is better than the other. To sum it up, deductive logic, the science of cause and effect, tends to view the world of matter in the dimension of time. Inductive logic sees a world of energy in the dimension of space. The universe is composed of matter and energy existing in space-time.

In the West, scientists applied deductive logic to successfully explain and classify matter that occupies space. Now the theoretical physicists are struggling to classify and understand energy; this is the quest for the Grand Unification Theory which attempts to unify the identified four fundamental forces: the strong force, the electroweak force, the electromagnetic force and eventually the force of gravity into a unified principle of energy.

Scientists in China studied and classified energy using inductive logic to successfully explain and classify energy by observing change (which takes time). They started with a unifying principle of energy called *yinyang* and struggled to understand matter. To them, matter was primarily 'packaged energy.' So we could specify colonqi, earthqi, heavenqi, cloudqi, snakeqi, rockqi, bananaqi, onionqi, humanqi, maleqi, femaleqi—even emptiness could be classified (a doorway has *Qi*). Chinese medical science uses over seventy terms for different types of energy.

Glossary of Terms in English

There are two types of definitions that follow:

Chinese dictionary definitions follow a number and Traditional Chinese Medicine (TCM) definitions follow TCM.

Acupoints are spots on the body known since ancient times to relieve pain and speed healing. When an acupoint or a pattern of acupoints is sore it can indicate problems elsewhere.

Blood (XUE 血 sounds like "shoe+way") 1: blood. In TCM it is a type of energy similar to blood as understood in the West, but Chinese medicine identifies more functions such as moistening tissue and nourishing the *Qi*. Blood can *congeal* and cause aching.

Body Inch (CUN 寸 sounds like "tsoon") 1: inch; 2: small. In TCM it is a unit of body measurement similar to an inch, but the actual distance varies from person to person. On an individual the *cun* varies depending on the body part.

Congealed Blood (YUXUE 瘀 血 sounds like "you shoe+way") 1: bruise; 2: poor circulation. In TCM *Congealed Blood* is an *excess* symptom pattern that appears when *Qi* energy pools and *blood congeals*. Relieve the pain by moving energy through the area. Felt as a dull ache, it accompanies or follows *Qi Stagnation (QIZHI)*. Palpable as ropy, stiff muscle.

Deficiency (XU 虚 sounds like "shoe") 1: void; 2: empty; 3: in vain; 4: timid; 5: false, deceitful; 6: humble, modest; 7: weakness, poor health; 8: theory; 9: virtual, facade. In TCM it is a symptom pattern indicating false health, characterized by degeneration of bodily functions, similar to chronic disease. Degeneration weakens the body and it loses the ability to eliminate *excess* during acute diseases.

Got Qi (Deqi 得氣 sounds like "duh chee") *DE* 1: to get, gain 2: suitable 3: compliant. In TCM *Deqi* (got *Qi)* is that healing feeling produced by stimulating acupoints, which *moves Qi (DAOQI)* energy. After gaining the desired *Qi* response, it may feel swollen, achy, numb and/or tingly, first locally then distant from the point of stimulation.

Energy (Qi 氣 sounds like "chee") 1: air, gas; 2: weather; 3: breath; 4: odor; 5: airs, manners; 6: spirited; 7: angry. In TCM it is the function of organs and systems referred to as the life force or bio-energy (function) of the organ. However, it is not energy as opposed to matter: neither is it energy like fuel.

Essence (JING 精 sounds like "jeeng") 1: refined, choice; 2: essence, extract; 3:spirit; 4: smart; 5: sperm. In TCM it is the material potential for growth similar to the genetic code. It originates at conception from the uniting of sperm and egg. *Qi* from food, supplements *JING;* likewise *JING* produces *Qi.* The quality of *JING* determines the quality of *Qi.*

Essential Energy (JINGQI 精氣 sounds like "jeeng chee") In TCM *Essential Qi* is the most material of *Qi* energy. *Qi* production consumes *JING.* This vital essence *JINGQI* is stored in the kidneys and regulates sexual energy, reproduction, growth and development including the aging process.

Excess (SHI 實 sounds like "sure") 1: solid; 2: true, real, honest; 3: fruit, seed. In TCM it is a symptom pattern indicating true health, characterized by discharge, similar to acute disease. Symptoms appear when the body eliminates microorganisms and toxins. The ability to eliminate *excess* degenerates with *deficiency* diseases (chronic).

Meridian (JING 經 sounds like "jeeng") 1: menses; 2: longitude; 3: pass through; 4: manage; 5: regular; 6: warp (in weaving) 7: classic book. In TCM it is a path on which *Qi* energy usually travels located between skin and bone. Stuck *Qi* energy in or near a path disrupts smooth bodily activity and results in pain. Acupoints on the skin provide access to these paths moving *Qi* energy *(DAOQI)* and relieve pain.

Move Qi (DAOQI 導氣 sounds like "dow chee") *DAO* 1: to lead; 2: to guide; 3: (in physics) to conduct. In TCM *Move Qi* means to move stuck or injured *Qi* energy, which assists the body to heal disease; thus: pain goes when energy flows. When *Qi* moves it may be experienced as *deqi (Got Qi)*.

Sedate (XIE 寫 sounds like "she+ah") 1: write; 2: draw, sketch. In TCM it is a therapeutic response used to release, reduce, disperse *excess Qi* energy

Shiatzu (The Japanese sounds like "she+ah tzoo"; the Chinese characters *ZHI* 指 *YA* 壓) a Japanese style massage used for pain relief, relaxation and medical therapy.

Stagnant Qi (QIZHI 氣滯 sounds like "chee jee") *ZHI* 1: stagnant; 2: stoppage; 3: junk. In TCM *Stagnant Qi* is blocked energy usually experienced as a sharp pain. An *excess* pattern appears when *Qi* energy pools at an acupoint, along a *meridian* or anywhere in the body it becomes "stuck." It is often the first stage of disease after *Qi* energy *stagnates,* the *blood* will *congeal* unless energy is moved through the area.

Tender Spot (AHSHI 阿是 sounds like "ahh sure") In TCM an *AHSHI* acupoint means the spot is tender when pressed. It guides a therapist in finding stuck and injured *Qi* energy. Ashi acupoints can form patterns that indicate a deep root.

Tonify (BU 補 sounds like "boo") 1: repair; 2: supply, fill; 3: nourish; 4: benefit. In TCM it is therapy to reinforce or strengthen *deficiency Qi* energy

Glossary of Terms in Pinyin

There are two types of definitions that follow:

Chinese dictionary definitions follow a number and Traditional Chinese Medicine (TCM) definitions follow TCM.

AHSHI (阿是 sounds like "ahh sure") In TCM an *AHSHI* acupoint means the spot is tender when pressed. It guides a therapist in finding stuck and injured *Qi* energy. Ashi acupoints can form patterns that indicate a deep root.

Anmo (按摩 sounds like "ahn Moe"). In TCM literally pressing (按) and rubbing (摩); the name of a therapy employed to *tonify* a *deficiency* of *Qi* energy. They are two of four basic movements used in *Shiatzu*.

BU (補 sounds like "boo"). 1: repair; 2: supply, fill; 3: nourish; 4: benefit. In TCM *BU (Tonify)* is therapy to reinforce or strengthen *deficiency Qi* energy

CUN (寸 sounds like "tsoon") 1: inch; 2: small. In TCM *Cun* is a unit of body measurement similar to an inch, but the actual distance varies from person to person. On an individual the *cun* varies depending on the body part.

DAOQI (導氣 sounds like "dow chee") *DAO* 1: to lead; 2: to guide; 3: (physics) to conduct. In TCM *DAOQI (Move Qi)* means to move stuck or injured *Qi* energy, which assists the body to heal disease; thus: pain goes when energy flows. When *Qi* moves it may be experienced as *deqi (Got Qi)*.

Deqi (Got Qi 得氣 sounds like "duh chee") *DE* 1: to get, gain 2: suitable 3: compliant. In TCM *Deqi* (got *Qi)* is that healing feeling produced by stimulating acupoints, which *moves Qi* (DAOQI) energy. After gaining the desired *Qi* response, it may feel swollen, achy, numb and/or tingly, first locally then distant from the point of stimulation.

JING (經 sounds like "jeeng") 1: menses; 2: longitude; 3: pass through; 4: manage; 5: regular; 6: warp (in weaving) 7: classic book. In TCM *JING (meridians)* is a path on which *Qi* energy usually travels located between skin and bone. *Stagnant Qi* energy in or near a path disrupts smooth bodily activity and results in pain. Acupoints on the skin provide access to these paths which *DAOQI (move Qi* energy) and relieve pain.

JING (精 sounds like "jeeng") 1: refined, choice; 2: essence, extract; 3:spirit; 4: smart; 5: sperm. In TCM *JING (Essence)* is the material potential for growth similar to the genetic code. It originates at conception from the uniting of sperm and egg. *Qi* from food, supplements *JING*; likewise *JING* produces *Qi*. The quality of *JING* determines the quality of *Qi*.

JINGQI (精氣 sounds like "jeeng chee") In TCM *JINGQI (Essential Qi)* is the most material of *Qi* energy. *Qi* production consumes *JING*. This vital essence *JINGQI* is stored in the kidneys and regulates sexual energy, reproduction, growth and development including the aging process.

Qi (氣 sounds like "chee") 1: air, gas; 2: weather; 3: breath; 4: odor; 5: airs, manners; 6: spirited; 7: angry. In TCM *Qi* energy is the function of organs and systems referred to as the life force or bio-energy (function) of the organ. However, it is not energy as opposed to matter; neither is it energy like fuel.

QIZHI (氣滯 sounds like "chee jee") *ZHI* 1: stagnant; 2: stoppage; 3: junk. In TCM *QIZHI (Stagnant Qi)* is blocked energy usually experienced as a sharp pain. An *excess* pattern appears when *Qi* energy pools at an acupoint, along a *meridian* or anywhere in the body it becomes 'stuck.' It is often the first stage of disease after *Qi* energy *stagnates*, the *blood* will *congeal* unless energy is moved through the area.

SHI (實 sounds like "sure") 1: solid; 2: true, real, honest; 3: fruit, seed. In TCM it is a symptom pattern indicating true health, characterized by discharge, similar to acute disease. Symptoms appear when the body eliminates microorganisms and toxins. The ability to eliminate *excess* degenerates with *deficiency* diseases (chronic).

Tuina (推拿 sounds like "two+we nah") In TCM literally stroking (推) and pinching (拿); the name of a therapy employed to disperse *excess Qi* energy. They are two of four basic movements used in *Shiatzu*.

XIE (寫 sounds like "she+ah") 1: write; 2: draw, sketch. In TCM *XIE (Sedate)* is a therapeutic response used to release, reduce, disperse *excess Qi* energy

XU (虛 sounds like "shoe") 1: void; 2: empty; 3: in vain; 4: timid; 5: false, deceitful; 6: humble, modest; 7: weakness, poor health; 8: theory; 9: virtual, facade. In TCM it is a symptom pattern indicating false health, characterized by degeneration of bodily functions, similar to chronic disease. Degeneration weakens the body and it loses the ability to eliminate *excess* during acute diseases.

XUE (血 sounds like "shoe+way") 1: blood. In TCM *XUE (Blood)* is a type of energy similar to blood as understood in the West, but Chinese medicine identifies more functions such as moistening tissue and nourishing the *Qi*. Blood can *congeal* and cause aching.

Yang (陽 sounds like "yah+ng"). In TCM and in the Chinese language yang is used as an adjective indicating the fiery, warming, drying nature of the modified word.

Yangqi (陽氣 sounds like "yah+ng chee"). In TCM it is the functional aspect of bio-energy; disease manifests as external, upward, hyperactive, inflammation and discharge.

Yin (陰 sounds like "y+een"). In TCM and in the Chinese language yin is used as an adjective indicating the watery, cooling, moistening nature of the modified word.

Yinqi (氣陰 sounds like "y+een chee"). In TCM it is the material aspect of bio-energy; disease manifests as *internal*, downward, hypoactive, weakness and congestion.

YUXUE (瘀血 sounds like "you shoe+way") *YU* 1:bruise; 2: poor circulation. In TCM *YUXUE (Congealed Blood)* is an *excess* symptom pattern, which appears when *Qi* energy pools and *blood congeals*. Relieve the pain by moving energy through the area. Felt as a dull ache, it accompanies or follows *Qi Stagnation (QIZHI)*. Palpable as ropy, stiff muscle.

Recommended Reading

"Food heals hunger; study heals ignorance."
"Gold is expensive; learning is priceless."
"Learning is like rowing upstream—advance or lose all."
    —Chinese proverbs

The interest in Asian healing arts has blossomed since I began writing this book. In my estimation, the following books are the finest in the field. Some are perennial best sellers and others, though in print, may be hard to find.

Acupressure's Potent Points, A Guide to Self-Care for Common Ailments
By Michael Reed Gach
Bantam Books
ISBN 0-553-34970-8
    Potent Points is a concise manual for the practical application of acupressure useful for the layman or professional. Each chapter covers a specific ailment including helpful acupoints, stretches and routines for alleviating problems varying from migraines to low back pain.

Basics Of Acupuncture, 4th Edition
By Gabriel Stux and Bruce Pomeranz
Springer-Verlag
ISBN 3-540-63235-2
    This is the only book on acupuncture published by a medical publishing house. It was written by medical educators for medical professionals. The scientist, Dr. Pomeranz, wrote a chapter for those interested in understanding the scientific basis of acupuncture, followed by a detailed account of the theory and practice of traditional Chinese medicine.

Do-It-Yourself Shiatsu
By Wataru Ohashi, Vicki Lindner (Editor)
Viking Penguin Books
ISBN 0-14-019351-0
www.ohashi.com

Ohashi is a pioneer in bringing *Shiatzu* to America. This book has served as required reading for my *Shiatzu* classes since its publication in 1976. It has never gone out of print. Included is a detailed description of over one hundred acupoints, and every chapter includes hints on how to successfully improve health and relieve the symptoms of disease.

The Gift Of Pain originally titled *Pain: the Gift Nobody Wants*
By Dr. Paul Brand and Philip Yancey
Zondervan Publishing House
ISBN 0-310-22144-7

I cannot say it better than C. Everett Koop who says Dr. Brand is "a surgeon, scholar, investigator and philosopher gifted with rare insight." This book does not advocate acupressure or other alternative means, but it is a "must read" for those suffering from chronic pain who want to understand and seek practical suggestions on dealing with pain.

Healing And The Mind
By Bill Moyers
Doubleday/Bantam Doubleday Dell Publishing Group, Inc.
ISBN 0-385-46870-9

The acclaimed television journalist Bill Moyers authors this book based on the ground-breaking video series which attempts to heal the rift between modern and ancient ideas of body and mind.

The Ohashi Bodywork Book
By Wataru Ohashi
ISBN 1-56836-096-7
www.ohashi.com

Ohashi is a true master of *Shiatsu* who has taken *Shiatsu* beyond tradition. He emphasizes mutual exchange of energy through bodywork that enriches both the giver and receiver. He reveals the secrets of his style, which have taken a lifetime to develop.

Spontaneous Healing
By Andrew Weil, M.D.
Borzoi Books
ISBN 0-679-43607-3

An inspirational book for those suffering from difficult health problems. Dr. Weil is an original thinker whose message is needed today. Acupuncture is one of many specific healing methods suggested in this book.

Thai Massage: A Traditional Medical Technique
By Richard Gold
Churchill Livingstone
ISBN 0-443-05935-7

This is the first book in English that I know of on Thai massage—another example of the influence of Chinese medicine. Richard Gold is a doctor of Oriental medicine and an educator who went to Thailand to study this unique massage style. This book is a practical guide with excellent visual aids.

*The Web That Has No Weaver, Understanding Chinese
    Medicine*
By Ted J. Kaptchuk, O.M.D.
Congdon & Weed, Inc.
ISBN 0-8092-2933-1

This vital classic explores deep concepts of Chinese medicine presented simply for the layman. Many acupuncture schools use this as a first year text.

The Yellow Emperor's Classic Of Medicine, The Essential Text of Chinese Health and Healing
By Maoshing Ni, Ph.D.
Shambhala
ISBN 1-57062-080-6
   Of the many translations, I think this one is the best over-all. The translator is a doctor of Oriental medicine and a licensed acupuncturist born into a family of medical practitioners that span many generations.

   For additional books about Oriental medicine, acupuncture and acupressure:

BLUE POPPY PRESS
(800) 487-9296
3450 Penrose Place, Ste. 110
Boulder, CO 80301
www.bluepoppy.com
Ask about these Blue Poppy recommended titles:
   The Curing Series (On topics including: PMS, fibromyalgia, depression, insomnia and more)
   Pediatric Massage
   The Tao Of Healthy Eating
   Blue Poppy publishes many excellent translations of medical classics.

REDWING BOOKS
(800) 873-3946
44 Linden St.
Brookline, MA 02445
www.redwingbooks.com
Ask about these Redwing recommended titles:
   Wood Becomes Water
   Who Can Ride The Dragon?
   Principles of Chinese Medicine
   Principles of Acupuncture

Recommended Schools

"Teachers open the door; you enter by yourself."
"A good teacher is better than a stack of books."
—Chinese proverbs

The following schools are recommended because I have known many graduates who thought highly of these schools and their teachers.

BOSTON SHIATSU SCHOOL
(617) 497-6630
1972 Mass Ave.
Cambridge, Massachusetts 02140
www.bostonshiatsu.org

HEARTWOOD INSTITUTE
(707) 923-5000
220 Harmony Lane
Garberville, CA 95542
www.heartwoodinstitute.com

MUELLER COLLEGE
(619) 291-9811
4607 Park Blvd.
San Diego, CA 92116
www.muellercollege.com

NATIONAL HOLISTIC INSTITUTE
(510) 547-6442
5900 Hollis St., Ste. J
Emeryville, CA 94608
www.nhimassage.com

OHASHI INSTITUTE
(518) 758-7404
P.O. Box 505
Kinderhook, NY 12106
www.ohashi.com

PACIFIC COLLEGE OF ORIENTAL MEDICINE
(619) 574-6909
3501 4th Ave.
San Diego, CA 92103
www.ormed.edu

OTHER SCHOOLS
Visit our Website at www.learnacupressure.com for updated additions to this list of recommended schools.

Bibliography
"A nation's treasure is its scholars."
—Chinese proverbs

Brand, Paul and Philip Yancey
1993 *Pain: The Gift Nobody Wants*, USA

Barber, Elizabeth Wayland
1999 *The Mummies of Ürümchi*, New York

Barnes, Gina L.
1993 *China, Korea and Japan: The Rise of Civilization in East Asia*, London

Catalano, E. and K. Hardin
1996 *The Chronic Pain Control Workbook*, USA

Chang Chi-yun
1962 *Chinese History of Fifty Centuries*, Taiwan

Chen, C. Y.
1969 *History of Chinese Medical Science Illustrated with Pictures*, Hong Kong

Chia, Mantak
1983 *Awaken Healing Energy Through The Tao*, USA

Deadman, Peter and Mazin Al-Khafaji
1998 *A Manual Of Acupuncture*, England

Ellis, Andrew and Nigel Wiseman and Ken Boss
1989 *Grasping the Wind*, Massachusetts, USA

Fenn, Courtenay H.
1969 *The Five Thousand Dictionary Chinese-English*, USA

Flaws, Bob
1994 *Statements of Fact in Traditional Chinese Medicine*, USA

Foreign Language Press
1980 *Essentials of Chinese Acupuncture*, Beijing

Hoizey, Dominique and Marie-Joseph
1993 *A History of Chinese Medicine*, Canada

Hsu, Hong-Yen and William G. Peacher
Chen's History Of Chinese Medical Science, Taiwan

Huang-fu Mi
1993 *The Systematic Classic of Acupuncture and Moxibustion*, Colorado, USA

Kaptchunk, Ted J.
1983 *The Web That Has No Weaver*, USA

Kessel, Joseph
1961 *The Man With The Miraculous Hands*, USA

Ki Sunu
1985 *The Canon of Acupuncture*, California

Koo, Linda Chih-ling
1982 *Nourishment of Life*, Quarry Bay, Hong Kong

Lade, Arnie
1989 *Acupuncture Points, Images and Functions*, Washington, USA

Lewis, C. S.
1962 *The Problem of Pain*, New York

Li Su Huai, translated by M. D. Broffman and Pei Sun F.
1976 *Points: 2001*, Kuan Tu, Taiwan

Liao, Sung J.
1983   *Chinese-English Terminology of Traditional Chinese Medicine,*

Liu, Frank and Liu Yan Mau
1980   *Chinese Medical Terminology,* Hong Kong

Lu, Henry C.
1978   *Nei Ching and Nan Ching,* Vancouver, Canada

Mather, Cotton
1972   *The Angel of Bethesda,* USA reprint

Melzack, Ronald
1973   *The Puzzle of Pain,* New York

Morris, David B.
1991   *The Culture of Pain,* USA

Moyers, Bill
1993   *Healing and the Mind,* New York

Needham, Joseph
1969-86   *Science and Civilization in China,* vol. 1-6, England

Ni, Maoshing, translation with commentary
1995   *The Yellow Emperor's Classic of Medicine,* USA

O'Connor, John and Dan Bensky
1981   *Acupuncture: A Comprehensive Text,* USA

Ohashi, Wataru
1976   *Do-it-Yourself Shiatsu,* New York

Ou Ming
1988   *Chinese-English Dictionary of Traditional Medicine,* Hong Kong

Porkert, Manfred
1974 *The Theoretical Functions of Chinese Medicine*, London

Reid, Daniel
1994 *The Complete Book of Chinese Health and Healing*, California

Shaughnessy, Edward L., translation and commentary
1996 *I Ching: The Classic of Changes*, New York

Shipley, Joseph T.
1945 *Dictionary of Word Origins*, New York

Sigerist, Henry E.
1951 *A History of Medicine*, vol. 1–2, New York

Sima Qian, and Burton Watson, translator
1961 *Records of the Grand Historian*, vol. 1–3, New York

Stux, Gabriel and Bruce Pomeranz
1998 *Basics of Acupuncture Fourth Edition*, New York

Temple, Robert
1986 *The Genius of China*, USA

Unschuld, Paul U.
1985 *Medicine in China; A History of Ideas*, California

Veith, Ilza, translated with introduction
1949 *The Yellow Emperor's Classic of Internal Medicine*, California

Ward, Milton
1977 *The Brilliant Function of Pain*, New York

Ware, J. R.
1966 *Alchemy, Medicine, Religion in the China of A.D. 320*, MIT, USA

Wieger, SJ, L.
1965 *Chinese Characters*, New York

Wilder, G. D. and J. H. Ingram
1974 *Analysis of Chinese Characters*, New York

Wilhelm, Richard
1950 *The I Ching or Book of Changes*, New York

Wiseman, Nigel
1995 *English-Chinese Dictionary of Chinese Medicine*, China

Wood, Ernest
1962 *A Study of Pleasure and Pain*, Illinois, USA

Wu Jing-Nuan
1993 *Ling Shu, (or) The Spiritual Pivot* Hawaii, USA

Wu, K.C.
1982 *The Chinese Heritage*, New York

Xie Zhufan and Huang Xiaokai, Editors
1984 *Dictionary of Traditional Chinese Medicine*, Hong Kong

Yates, Robin D. S.
1997 *Five Lost Classics: Tao, Huanglao, and Yin-yang in Han China*, New York

Zhou Chuncai
1996 *The Yellow Emperor's Medicine Classic*, Singapore

Afterword

"Many words; some mistakes."
—Chinese proverb

The words and translations contained in this book are my own. No standard English translation of terms has been established in Traditional Chinese Medicine (TCM).

TCM is at least two thousand five hundred years old and possibly four thousand years old. It has been proven effective today. The scientist and professor, Bruce Pomeranz, M.D., Ph.D., has discovered and published over fifty articles in peer review journals, proving that acupuncture works for relieving pain. The best way to make it work is debatable. Many traditions have appeared in the last two millennia.

Many of the theories, ideas and terms published in this book may be disputed by other successful healers and scholars. The reasons for this are: 1) the fine points of TCM have been disputed for two millennia in China, 2) TCM is a product of Chinese thinking, and in the process of translating the terms and ideas into other languages many disputes have arisen, and 3) I have changed my ideas as I've continued to learn. For example, today in China, more articles have been published on "What is the Sanjiao (Triple Heater)?" than on any other subject. Also, numerous translation difficulties can be observed by simply consulting a number of English translations of Chinese texts. The term *PI* has been translated as spleen, which functions as the 'master organ of digestion.' Therefore, many TCM scholars now agree that the organ *PI* should be translated as pancreas, yet no book uses this term. Only a few use the term spleen-pancreas. Many controversies remain. However, as far as I know, all schools agree pain is injured (blocked) *Qi* and, to remove pain, *Qi* must flow.

Many other examples could be given, but this book is not about resolving problems of scholarship. It is about solving the problem of pain. There is no dispute acupuncture and acupressure, when applied appropriately, can reduce and relieve pain. However, many terms are discussed and the choice of the translated terms and what they mean are solely my own. If you disagree with my translations or ideas, you are invited to tell me why you disagree. I want to feel free to change my mind as I gain new knowledge and insight regarding my understanding of TCM and the Chinese culture that produced it. Finally, the proof of a theory is the result it produces. Great theories may not work. Many a beautiful theory has been destroyed by an ugly fact.

All healing, East and West, has as its goal the alleviation of human suffering. I sincerely hope this book helps to bridge the conflicting ideologies that exist and benefits those suffering from pain.

E-mail me at acupress@learnacupressure.com.

Index

Acupoint IDs

Acupoint Names

Books and Classics

Nations and Nationalities

America: -11, -2, 29, 137

Anyang: 32, 38, 42, 161

Asia (Far East, Oriental): -11, 26, 29 *ff.*, 51 *ff.*, 59–60, 70, 137, 168–70

Bactria: 169

Beijing (Peking): 38

Belgium: 4–5

Caucasian: 169–70

China (中國 Zhongguo): -4 *ff.*, 10–3, 29 *ff.*, 44 *ff.*, 50 *ff.*, 104, 160–3, 167–70, 242

Denmark: 4

Dutch: 4–5

France: 4–5

Great Yuezhi (Tocharian): 47, 168–9

Greece: 34

Han (寒): 30–4, 38–40, 50

Henan: 38

Himalayan: 47

Hindu (India): 2, 35

Holland: 4–5

Huns: 40, 168–9

India (Hindu): 2, 35

Japanese: -1, 25, 53–4, 114

Koreans: 47, 53, 60

Macedonia: 34

Norway: 4

Persia: 34

Poland: 4

Qin (秦): 30, 33–4, 39, 47–50

Rome: 34

Russian Turkestan: 169

Shang (商): 30–2, 34, 38–34, 49, 59, 161, 168

Silk Road: 168–9

Sumeria: 35

Tarim Basin: 47, 169

Tibet: 3, 47, 53, 169

Tocharian (Great Yuezhi): 47, 168–9

Turkic speaking: 168

Vietnamese: 47, 53

Wei River: 32–3, 46–7

Xia (夏): 30–1, 39

Yellow River (黄河 Huanghe): -3, 11, 31–3, 38, 46–7, 60, 104, 169

Yugoslavia: 4

Zhou (周): 30, 32–9, 42, 45–7, 49, 59, 162

People and Professions

Pinyin (English) Terms

TCM Terms English (Pinyin)

networking channel (絡脈 luomai): 107

numbness (麻 ma): 22, 84–5

original *Qi* (元氣 yuanqi): 13, 183

pain (痛 tong): 8–10, 19 *ff.*, 54, 70 *ff.*, 102, 119, 176, 199, 238–40

penetrating wind: 138

pinch (拿 na): 81, 87–90, 200 *ff.*

press (摩 mo): 81, 87–9, 102, 200 *ff.*

produce (生 sheng): 13, 14

pulse, Chinese (脈 mai): 51

pulse temple: 165

quality (虛實 xushi): 66–9, 76–9

Roots and Branches, theory of: 72, 74

rub (按 an): 81, 87–8, 102, 200 *ff.*

scholar (士 shi): 32–3, 36–41, 48–9, 162–3, 189

sea of Blood: 178

sea of marrow: 135, 158

sea of nutrition: 115

sedate (瀉 xie): 73, 84–5, 245, 248

skeletal system gathering: 178

source (原 yuan): 107

spirit bright, enlightened thinking (神明 shenming): 236, 238

spirit (神 shen): 14, 236, 238

stagnant Qi (氣滯 qizhi): 18, 24, 52, 86, 174, 71, 243, 245, 247, 249

stroke (推 tui): 81, 87–90, 200 *ff.*

sun (太陽 taiyang): 165 *ff.*

tender spot(阿是 ahshi): 245, 246

tonify (補 bu): 73, 84–5, 245, 246

upper energy point: 153

water (水 shui): 51, 62–4, 98–9

wind (風 feng): 74, 99, 137–8, 158

wind heat: 138

windows of heaven: 147

yang(陽): 57, 60 *ff.*, 100–1, 112, 165–70, 181, 238–40, 248

yin(陰): 57, 60 *ff.*, 100–1, 109, 112, 168–70, 181, 238–40, 248

yinyang(陰陽): 45–6, 51, 57 *ff.*, 233–4, 238–40

General